The Successful GP Re Companion

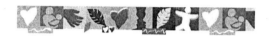

Library & Information Services

Airedale **NHS**
NHS Trust

For Churchill Livingstone:

Commissioning Editor: Heidi Allen
Development Editor: Robert Edwards
Project Manager: Derek Robertson
Design Direction: George Ajayi

The Successful GP Registrar's Companion

Preparing, practising and perfecting

Edited by

Joe Rosenthal BSC MSC MBBCh DRCOG FRCGP DFFP
Senior Lecturer in General Practice, Royal Free & University College Medical School, London, UK

Jeannette Naish MSC MBBS FRCGP
Senior Lecturer in General Practice, Queen Mary's School of Medicine & Dentistry, London, UK

Surinder Singh BM MSC DRCOG FRCGP DGM ILTM
Clinical lecturer in General Practice, Royal Free & University College Medical School, London, UK

Roger Neighbour MA MB BChir DRCOG FRCGP
General Practitioner, Abbots Langley, Hertfordshire

Foreword by
John Toby CBE FRCP FRCGP
Chairman of the Joint Committee for Postgraduate Training in General Practice, Royal College of General Practitioners, London, UK

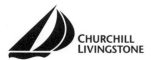
CHURCHILL
LIVINGSTONE

EDINBURGH LONDON NEW YORK OXFORD PHILADELPHIA ST LOUIS SYDNEY TORONTO 2003

CHURCHILL LIVINGSTONE
An imprint of Elsevier Science Limited

ISBN 0 443 07225 6

British Library Cataloguing in Publication Data
A catalogue record for this book is available from the British Library

Library of Congress Cataloging in Publication Data
A catalog record for this book is available from the Library of Congress

Note
Medical knowledge is constantly changing. As new information becomes available,
changes in treatment, procedures, equipment and the use of drugs become necessary.
The editors, contributors and the publishers have taken care to ensure that the
information given in this text is accurate and up to date. However, readers are strongly
advised to confirm that the information, especially with regard to drug usage, complies
with the latest legislation and standards of practice.

your source for books,
journals and multimedia
in the health sciences
www.elsevierhealth.com

The
publisher's
policy is to use
**paper manufactured
from sustainable forests**

Printed in China

Contents

Examiners' Points appearing throughout the chapters are provided by Dr Roger Neighbour, former Convenor of the MRCGP Panel of Examiners

Contributors

Steve Gillam   General Practitioner, Luton
Director of Primary Care, King's Fund, London, UK
Public Health Course Director, University of Cambridge, UK
Visiting Professor University of Luton, UK

Margaret Lloyd   General Practitioner, London
Professor of Primary Care, Department of Primary Care & Population
Sciences, Royal Free & University College Medical School, London, UK

Hilary Scott   Deputy Health Service Ombudsman for England and Wales

Dee Stenning   Primary Care Computing Training & Development Co-ordinator, South
East London Shared Services Partnership. Former practice manager

Foreword

The predecessor of this Companion rapidly became a valued resource for GP registrars and their trainers. However, society, the world of general practice and its academic base have moved on. This is a time of change, with potentially bewildering possibilities and opportunities for those in training. GPs will work within more diverse situations in the future and they are increasingly applying the values and skills of the medical generalist in settings other than the traditional context of a conventional GP partnership. The continuing success of general practice and primary care will depend on maintaining these values and skills and making them the foundation for newly evolving pathways of care for patients. This makes the education of GPs a matter of even greater importance for the future and emphasizes the need for broadly based texts to guide them.

Education for general practice is also changing and will continue to do so as the impact of changes in the regulation, organisation and content of medical education as a whole are felt. However, learners will still make the transition into general practice. They, and their trainers, will still look for assistance in helping them to reorientate themselves and to make the best use of the learning opportunities that general practice provides. They will find these here.

The expanded editorial team and their contributors have brought a breadth of vision embracing anthropological, ethical and organisational perspectives as well as giving new insights from more traditional ones without losing sight of the central concern. As one might expect from these individuals, there remains a steady focus on the nature and role of the consultation, the relationships with patients and how these may be understood.

Society and the profession are rightly putting a greater emphasis on the quality of doctors, who require a wide range of skills as well as appropriate attitudes and the necessary knowledge. The techniques for ensuring high quality practice are explored but much depends on the personal approach of the doctor. The emphasis on the MRCGP examination and the assistance that it gives to potential candidates is therefore welcome.

But this is not a book that is solely about passing an examination; it offers insights into learning and teaching to help Registrars to develop themselves and points the way to topics for further discussion and sources to help inform those discussions.

I congratulate the editors, the contributors and their publishers on developing this new Companion which, I am sure, will occupy the same leading role in GP education in the future as its predecessor has done for a previous generation of Registrars.

2003   John Toby

Preface

This book follows in the footsteps of *The Trainee's Companion to General Practice*, originally published by Churchill Livingstone in 1994 and aimed at guiding the novice GP through the transition from hospital medicine to primary health care. Like its predecessor, this new *Successful Registrar's Companion* provides practical advice on the day-to-day work of the GP and the primary healthcare team, as well as exploring the fundamental principles that underpin this practice. Since the publication of the original book both general practice and education for general practice have been through significant change. All doctors should now be qualifying with greater awareness of primary care as a result of the increased exposure to the community in their undergraduate medical education; GP trainees are now renamed GP Registrars and summative assessment is a fact of their lives; the MRCGP exam has evolved a modular approach and novel training schemes are being developed and piloted. The NHS has celebrated its golden jubilee and has itself much changed. New models for providing primary care services both in and out of hours are emerging. The explicit recognition of 'quality' has become part of all GPs' work, through the introduction of clinical governance with its component elements such as audit, evidence-based practice and risk management. Medical ethics and law have moved from somewhere near the back to the forefront of doctors' and patients' minds, and a new contract proposing fundamental changes in the organisation of GP services is reaching the late stages of negotiation. To cap it all, compulsory revalidation of all doctors is on the near horizon. Related to all of these changes, information technology and electronic communication have had real impact on how most of us live, work and learn.

But some things have not changed The heart of general practice, the core activity in our view, remains the same now as when the NHS began in 1948. In the privacy of the consulting room, patients of any age, sex or background bring to us their health concerns of any kind. We listen, discuss, reassure, advise and help them to the best of our ability, making no financial demand upon them and using whatever resources we have available to us.

We have in this book attempted to keep this core activity in mind while covering all the main areas likely to concern the GP currently in training. The scope of general practice is boundless and no book can attempt to provide adequate coverage of all aspects of the discipline.

We have therefore concentrated on the areas of recent change as outlined above. We have consciously omitted discussion of the diagnosis and management of specific clinical problems, which we know is adequately covered in several other texts. What we offer is a set of self-contained 'bite-size' chapters that can be read in sequence or dipped into at different stages. Each of the chapters could be used as the basis of a trainer/registrar tutorial and all will be helpful in preparing for summative assessment and the MRCGP.

Two of the three lead editors (JR and JN) remain from the original Trainee's Companion. Margaret Lloyd is still one of our main contributors by way of three new ethics and law chapters. We are delighted to be joined on the editorial team by Surinder Singh and Roger Neighbour, both bringing welcome new dimensions to the book; Surinder, with his rare combination of training in both general practice and medical anthropology, and Roger, a 'GP celebrity' renowned for his work in general practice communication and vocational training, with his insider knowledge of the MRCGP as a recent Convenor of the examination. As well as contributing two vital chapters for any registrar to read, Roger has provided the series of 'Examiners' Points', which are scattered liberally throughout the book. These are intended to guide MRCGP candidates as to some of the particular issues upon which they would be well advised to reflect in their preparation and revision for the examination. We are grateful also to our other contributors – Steve Gillam, Hilary Scott and Dee Stenning – for sharing with us their expertise and insights, and to those registrars and colleagues who have read and commented on the material. Thanks as well must go to Ellen Green, Lynn Watt, Heidi Allen and Robert Edwards of Elsevier Science, who have steered the book through to publication.

For both GP Registrar and trainer this book should provide a framework upon which to build to make the very most of the opportunities of the Registrar year. We hope that it will also be of interest to any established GP as part of the constant task of keeping up-to-date with current thinking and looking critically at our work. Whoever reads this book, we hope above all that it will help you to enjoy the enormous stimulation and rich variety which is offered by a career in general practice.

London 2003

Joe Rosenthal
Jeannette Naish

SECTION 1 The registrar year

1 Getting the most out of your registrar year

Joe Rosenthal

The experience of medical education and training is peppered with memorable events. For the future GP, the year as a registrar in a training practice represents a major transitional stage in your career and a time you will always remember. As a junior doctor in hospital you will have usually worked with a very clearly defined role in a particular specialty. You will have learned to make decisions but not taken ultimate responsibility for patients' management or the organisation of the service in which you play your role. As a GP, although still working with a team, you must now learn to become a fully independent practitioner, responsible for your own patients and the smooth running of the practice as a whole. This chapter aims to help you to plan ahead and make the most of this important stage in your training by outlining the form and content of the GP registrar year and making some suggestions as to how best to approach it.

Until recent years, many doctors arrived at their GP registrar post with very minimal previous exposure to general practice and primary care other than perhaps a short GP placement as a medical student. However, following changing patterns of health care and recommendations by the General Medical Council (GMC) in 1993, all UK medical schools have increased the time that undergraduates spend in the community during their courses and so the general practice environment is becoming more familiar to doctors graduating at the beginning of the twenty-first century.

L The GMC reminds us that *all* doctors have teaching responsibilities. Even early in your career you could be called upon to teach attached medical students, receptionists or nursing colleagues. What lessons or experiences of your own might you want to pass on to them? Why might they not have learned them elsewhere already? What would be good ways to set up effective learning opportunities?

Some of you might even have undertaken one of a small but increasing number of pre-registration house officer posts that include a 4-month general practice component. This is progress, but the fact remains that the hospital setting is where you will have spent most of your time so far in medicine, and the move from hospital senior house officer to GP registrar represents a very big change. Almost everything in general practice is different from in hospital. Attitudes, hours of work, daily routines, patients' problems and expectations, paperwork and relationships with colleagues will all seem new. It is because of this different culture and type of work that the requirement of a year with individual supervision from an experienced GP trainer was devised in the early 1970s and became compulsory in 1979. Before that time, any fully registered doctor was eligible to take up a post as a GP within the National Health Service.

L Consider keeping a log of how things differ between primary and secondary care. Concentrate especially on contrasting ways of thinking, such as the differences between inductive and hypothesis-testing methods of problem-solving; how and why the traditional medical model has evolved in the GP context; how time is used differently; how systems of control and lines of accountability are different.

This brings us on to a brief look at the regulations for training as a GP. At the time of writing, the Vocational Training Regulations are under review and so it is important to check the up-to-date rules either with your local Department of Postgraduate GP Education or with the Joint Committee on Postgraduate Training in General Practice (JCPTGP), based at the Royal College of General Practitioners (website: www.rcgp.org.uk). The Department of Health (2000) also produces a guide on GP training in the UK, which can be found at www.doh.gov.uk/medicaltrainingintheuk/manual.htm. Until this review, the regulations remained largely unchanged since their 1979 introduction, apart from some small adjustments to bring them into line with EU legislation in 1994 and, more importantly, the introduction of summative assessment in 1997. The current general requirement is that, following house jobs, 1 year must be spent in hospital senior house officer posts approved from a list of specialties (see Box 1.1) and approved by the specialist Royal College, a further 1 year in any approved training post (this is almost invariably another year of hospital senior house officer training) and 1 year that must be spent as a registrar in

Box 1.1
Specialties usually approved for GP training at senior house officer level

- General medicine
- Geriatric medicine
- Paediatrics
- Psychiatry
- General surgery or A & E, or A & E with general surgery, or A & E with orthopaedics
- Obstetrics or gynaecology, or Obstetrics and gynaecology

an approved training practice. Only once you have acquired the necessary experience and successfully completed all aspects of summative assessment can you apply for your JCPTGP certificate of 'prescribed' or 'equivalent' experience, which is an essential requirement to practise as an unsupervised GP in the NHS whether in partnership, or as an assistant, locum or deputy.

Although these regulations have served general practice well, there is a widespread feeling amongst contemporary GP educators and professional bodies that they are now outdated, and there is much debate about developing a new training model that is more appropriate to the needs of future GPs. A number of pilot schemes are already in place, with innovative senior house officer rotations and extended or additional GP registrar posts.

Choosing a practice

However the regulatory framework develops, the importance of the registrar period will remain paramount and getting the most out of it might well depend on choosing the right practice and the right trainer to suit your own individual needs. Even if you are undergoing your training as part of a Vocational Training Scheme (VTS) package, you are likely to have some choice as to which practice you join as a registrar. Even if your scheme has allocated you to a practice, you should certainly visit, meet the trainer and ask yourself if it is the right placement for you. If you have doubts, try to define them clearly and then explore with your Course Organiser early on the areas of concern and, if necessary, discuss the possibility of changing. The most important issues in choosing a practice revolve around the relationship with your trainer and the balance offered between education and service. The system of trainer/practice selection and reapproval (usually every 3 years) should guarantee that any approved training practice will provide a sound experience, but there will naturally be a range of quality and styles to be found. Many trainees are concerned about geographical location; this is obviously an important consideration but it should not be an overriding one because the post is usually for 1 year only and the right practice will be worth travelling to, within reason.

In the past, a glance at the appointments section of any edition of the *British Medical Journal* (*BMJ*) would reveal a selection of GP registrar posts being advertised individually. Since April 2000, however, funding and administrative arrangements have changed and now the advertising and recruitment for all posts is done synchronously throughout the UK twice each year. The adverts appear in the *BMJ*, on the Department of Health website (www.doh.gov.uk/) and on each Region's Department of Postgraduate GP Education website. Shortlisting and interviews are managed by the Regional Deaneries and, once selected for training, the potential registrars are usually directed to locality trainers' groups for matching to practices. The system is designed to be open and based on equal opportunities. This centralised appointment system does not mean that choice is taken away from candidates. You should still start thinking about your placement in good time, give careful consideration to the type of practice you want and do some research about the training practices available in your chosen area. If there are particular practices that interest you then approach the trainer or practice manager and ask if you can visit. Try also to speak to the current or recent registrars from the practice. Here are some of the main issues that you should consider in your choice of practice.

■ **Type of practice** – large, small, inner city, suburban or rural? If you are fairly sure about the type of practice and sort of area where you want to eventually work then it makes sense to seek a training practice that fits with your long-term plans. Try to keep an open mind, however, as ideas about general practice conceived before training will often change as you learn more about the specialty.

> **L** Remember that the MRCGP exam will ask questions about all kinds and conditions of practice in the UK. Reflect on how things might be different in practices in other parts of the country, or of different size, demography and ethnic mix.

■ **Trainer's educational approach** – do you feel comfortable with the trainer's description of how he or she will approach the role with respect to your training, and also how you will be expected to approach meeting your learning needs? Ask particularly about any gaps you feel need filling in your knowledge or skills, and also how the tutorial programme is run. It is also worth exploring the trainer's views on how summative assessment needs are incorporated into the programme for the year. Ask if the practice has an introductory booklet or pack for registrars, as this could provide a good feel to how the registrar fits into the practice.

> **L** Check out your trainer's views about the MRCGP. Registrars whose trainers have a positive attitude towards the exam and keep themselves well-informed about it do significantly better than others, especially in the video module.

■ **Clinical experience** – does the practice population provide the mix of clinical experience you feel you are looking for? Is the workload large and broad enough to provide you with good clinical experience but not so heavy that you will find it difficult to reflect and learn? Ask to see an example of a trainee's weekly timetable and don't forget to discuss the on-call duties (both daytime and out of hours) that the registrar is expected to undertake.

■ **Educational resources** – is there an up-to-date library, internet access, video recorder and camera. Is there potential for exposure to learning experiences outside the practice?

■ **Financial/contractual considerations** – as a registrar you are employed by your training practice. Ask if they use the standard contract recommended by the Department of Health and British Medical Association (BMA) (available on line via www.doh.gov.uk/medicaltrainingintheuk). You can also read about the details of how registrars are paid in the Statement of Fees and allowances generally known as 'the Red Book' (Department of Health and Welsh Office 2002). This explains how your registrar salary relates to your most recent hospital post and covers issues such as removal expenses, car allowance and so on. It can be viewed on line at www.nhs.uk/redbook/

Phases of the registrar year

Try to think of your registrar year as a whole rather than just taking each day as it comes. Roger Neighbour's book *The Inner Apprentice* (Neighbour 1992) was written starting with the question of what makes the difference between fulfilling and underachieving GP traineeships. If you read this book you will gain valuable insights to help you get the very most out of the whole experience.

Pereira Gray (1977) has described the training year as having five phases (Table 1.1). During the year the registrar should develop independence and the tendency to practise hospital style medicine should give way to a sense of identity as a GP. Some training schemes divide the 12 months of practice attachment into two periods, with 1–6 months taking place at the beginning of the programme and the remainder at the end – after hospital posts – but the principle of travelling through these types of phases will still apply.

Table 1.1
Phases of the training year

Phase	Time scale	Change in registrar
Preparation	Before starting and first week	Registrar dependence
Adjustment	First month	Registrar has hospital outlook
Working	2–7 months	
Partnership	8–10 months	Registrar has developed GP outlook
Final	10–12 months	Trainee autonomy

Preparation phase   As the time to start the new post approaches, a little time can usefully be invested in some reading around the general practice literature (see the Further reading and sources of information section at the end of this book). Most medical libraries will hold copies of free publications such as *Pulse, GP* and *Doctor*, and you can get onto their mailing lists by phoning the circulation departments listed in each one. Also, by becoming an Associate of the Royal College of General Practitioners you can receive the *British Journal of General Practice* each month. By browsing through such material you can start to 'acclimatise' to the sorts of issues that are current both clinically and politically. The preparation phase continues into the first week or two of joining the practice, when you will be introduced to your new colleagues and the way the practice works. At this time, if you are joining a new group, you should also be getting to know your half-day release colleagues and course organiser.

> **L** Making the acquaintance of the RCGP at an early stage (e.g. by becoming an associate member) will help you get a feel for its values and the role it might play in your professional life, and hence help you decide whether to sit the membership exam.

Adjustment phase   It takes around a month for a new registrar to adjust to working in primary care. At the beginning of this induction period, you and your trainer will start to get to know each other and agree how you will work together. You will discuss your learning needs for the year and usually prepare a learning contract and a timetable, which will include plans for all the elements of your summative assessment (MCQ, audit, video and trainer's report). You will sit in on consultations with your trainer and other doctors in the practice and accompany them on home visits. You will start to observe your trainer dealing with the practice computer system, paperwork and administration in order to learn about the different systems, forms and procedures with which you must become familiar. You will spend time observing patients in the waiting area, helping reception staff and shadowing other members of the primary care team in both the practice and the community (e.g. district nurse, health visitor, midwife, community mental health team, palliative care team). A visit to the Primary Care Trust will help you understand how national and local services are organised. Meetings with the local pharmacist, social services and other community contacts (e.g. hospice, alcohol and drug services, undertaker) can be arranged during this time. You should also have the chance to shadow a doctor from the practice providing out-of-hours care by telephone, at an out-of-hours centre and/or on home visits, depending on local arrangements.

These first weeks are also a good time to get to know the local geography and start to build a list of useful contacts. The practice will supply a basic telephone list but you can personalise this as the year goes on.

Box 1.2
The registrar's basic equipment needs

Stethoscope, otoscope/ophthalmoscope, sphygmomanometer, thermometer, peak flow meter, patella hammer, torch, tongue depressors, gloves, KY jelly, tourniquet, blood and urine bottles, needles, syringes, urine and blood testing strips.

Paperwork and drugs required should be discussed with your trainer.

You will also be building up your own set of medical equipment and supplies (Box 1.2) in discussion with your trainer.

After the intense activity of junior hospital posts, this observational role might sound rather passive, but this need not be the case if you look upon this period as the foundation for the year ahead. Use it as an opportunity to learn actively about the way primary health care works and to form relationships with colleagues with whom you will be working closely in the future. To balance the observational role of the adjustment phase it is a good idea to start to see a few patients in mini-surgeries. Receptionists will be asked to book patients at initially longer intervals and your trainer will be available to discuss any questions that you might have during or after each surgery. At first you might feel overwhelmed with uncertainties about how to manage different and often unfamiliar sorts of problems, which forms to use, how to enter data on the computer, when and where to get advice or refer.

Many registrars find it helpful to start a 'learning journal' at this stage. This can be kept in a book or on a PC or handheld computer. At its simplest, it could be a log diary of the events of each day. However, the idea can be taken much further if the journal is used as a reflective record not just of what you have seen and done but also of how you felt about and what you have gained from each new experience.

In these first weeks you will learn a great deal in a short time and will realise early-on that you can deal effectively with most of the problems that present to you. Soon you will start to feel like a GP.

The adjustment phase of the registrar year (first month)

- Agree learning contract, including plans for summative assessment
- Plan timetable, including surgeries, tutorials and half-day release
- Get to know the practice doctors and other clinical and administrative staff
- Get to know the local geography
- Observe the waiting area and reception during surgery time
- Sit in on consultations
- Get familiar with computing and administrative systems
- Visit local pharmacists, social services, Primary Care Trust, etc.
- Start building a list of useful contacts

- Start a 'learning journal'
- Collect equipment for bag
- Observe out-of-hours arrangements
- Start mini-surgeries
- Do some background reading

Working phase   The essence of this phase is learning by doing and assessing progress. After the first 2–4 weeks you will start to run your own regular surgeries. Most established GPs book patients at 10-min intervals. As a new registrar you will initially be booked with longer slots while you settle in; 20 min is probably a reasonable time to start with but remember that this luxury is only temporary and you will have to learn to find ways of managing time to fit in with the demands of real-life general practice. If you have worked in hospital outpatient clinics or casualty departments you will already be familiar with seeing patients at speed but still being both caring and thorough. This is a fundamental skill in any branch of clinical medicine but what is different in general practice is the huge variety of problems that can come through your door in any one surgery. You need to learn to switch from cardiologist to gynaecologist to geriatrician to counsellor and so on in quick succession. For most GPs this is the thrill of the job and after a time we don't think in terms of the category of the problem but the personality and needs of the patient. To cope with the pace and range of patient contacts we all need to evaluate what we can offer to patients with any particular problem. As well as knowledge of theory and evidence, we also need a lot of practice seeing large numbers of patients to gain the experience we need as a grounding for our application of knowledge.

Reception staff should inform patients when they book to see you that you are a new registrar in the practice and this might influence the sort of people you see initially. Some may be directed by your trainer, some may have seen your predecessor, some may be just curious to meet the new doctor and some may see you just because you have the shortest waiting time. This is a good time to discuss with your trainer how you decide which patients to bring back to your own surgeries and which to advise to return to their regular doctor if they have one. As a general rule, the default position should be that those patients whom you see for whatever reason and who require subsequent follow-up should come back to you if they are happy to do so. If you merely see snapshots of patients' problems and then send them back to another doctor in the practice you will miss out on many valuable learning opportunities. Don't be shy to ask patients to come back and see you for review so that you can see for yourself if they have got better following your initial advice or treatment. In this way you will learn by experience which problems resolve themselves and which treatments are more or less effective. Note down any questions that come to mind during your surgeries so that you can raise them afterwards with your trainer or look them up while they are fresh in your mind.

The appointment of a new doctor in any practice is an opportunity for a review of medical care. It is well known that a new pair of 'clinical eyes' can sometimes identify new diagnoses and solutions. Whereas established GPs will have a vast experience to share with you, it could also be the case that you are more up-to-date with certain aspects of medicine, which you have covered recently in the specialist hospital setting. Beware of the temptation to try and 'score points' by seeking new diagnoses and cures and remember that you and your trainer can learn from each other.

After the first 2 weeks of doing your own surgeries it is important to feel that you are seeing a full range of patients and problems. As a new doctor you will probably at first see a disproportionate amount of 'extras' – people with acute and often minor illness who wish to see the first available doctor. It is important to gain skills in managing such consultations but you also need a mixture of chronic disease management and health promotion work.

> **L** Having plenty of time to address relatively undemanding problems will allow you to think about other goals for the consultation. (See, for instance, the Stott and Davies model in Chapter 4, p. 46.) Developing a 'what else?' mind-set is good practice for the MRCGP written paper.

Your trainer will be able to introduce you to some patients with chronic diseases whom you can follow during the year. Involvement with health promotion and disease prevention can be arranged according to the practice set-up. The practice nurses often take the lead in running baby clinics, diabetic and antenatal clinics, all of which you should spend time in. If you are a female doctor in a practice where male doctors outnumber female then you might see a disproportionate amount of women and children. Discuss the balance of your clinical workload with your trainer and the receptionists if you feel it is not quite even.

During the working phase of the year, your summative assessment should be taking shape (see Chapter 2). You will need to have made a decision whether you plan to sit the exam to become a Member of the Royal College of General Practitioners (MRCGP) (this is optional, see Chapter 3) in addition to undergoing summative assessment (which is compulsory) because the multiple choice questions (MCQ) and video submission for MRCGP can also be used for summative assessment purposes. You should have prepared for, and taken, the MCQ, got underway with your audit and practised video-recording surgeries (see Chapters 2 and 3 on summative assessment and the MRCGP examination). Remember that summative assessment is a test of minimal competence, that is, it exists to identify the weakest 3–5% of registrars, whereas MRCGP is a test of excellence.

> **The working phase of the registrar year (months 2–7)**
>
> - Regular surgeries with decreasing appointment times
> - Home visits
> - Keep a list of patients seen
> - Monitor and discuss the case-mix you are seeing to ensure balance
> - Prepare for summative assessment/MRCGP MCQ
> - Prepare for summative assessment video submission (after month 6)
> - Prepare summative assessment written work
> - Work with trainer in reviewing knowledge, skills and attitudes
> - Raise problem cases or topics in tutorials
> - Make the most of your half-day release
> - Keep reading

Partnership phase   Usually by the third or fourth month the registrar is beginning to feel much more confident in the role of GP. His or her approach will have changed from that of a hospital doctor to a different style of managing patients and working with colleagues. At the same time, however, the novelty of being a GP can wear off, and surgeries begin to appear repetitive and paperwork tedious. Patients seem to present with insoluble problems and some do not improve in spite of your best efforts. In short, the honeymoon period is over and at this point the registrar's morale can slump. Remember at this point that no job is without aspects that are repetitive or difficult. It is important to try and identify precisely which aspects of the job you find difficult and to discuss them with your trainer and your half-day release group. Some problems will always be hard but others might get easier with experience and with help and advice from others who have to deal with the same issues.

As your confidence and competence grow in this part of the year, your relationship with your trainer will change. In the early part of the year the trainer has been the dominant, even parental figure in the relationship. During the 'partnership phase' the relationship moves closer to that of colleagues or partners and, although assessment continues, the registrar usually becomes more active in identifying areas of need and their solutions. The registrar might suggest that teaching arrangements are changed or that he or she attends particular courses, or perhaps might feel more need to discuss his or her problems outside the practice; it is now that the half-day release often takes on more importance. The registrar might also find that he or she is taking issue with some of the trainer's ideas and methods about clinical care and about practice organisation. These are all healthy developments in the educational process.

During the second half of the year the registrar should be directing his or her learning slightly less at clinical matters and more at practice organisational and management issues. Theoretically, after the registrar year you should be ready to take up a post as a GP Principal and take a full part in running a practice. It is therefore essential that you do gain a basic understanding of all aspects of practice management under the guidance of your trainer and the practice management staff. Some of your tutorial time will be spent on management topics and you will be able to do background reading, but it is also important to shadow the relevant staff members at work and to attend practice business meetings, staff meetings, finance meetings and partners' meetings whenever possible.

The partnership phase of the registrar year (months 8–10)

- Build up speed, confidence and competence in managing patients in surgery
- Work with some 'challenging patients'
- Work on identified areas of weakness
- Concentrate more on practice administration and management
- Make the most of tutorials and half-day release
- Submit summative assessment video or sit simulated surgery
- Submit summative assessment written work
- Keep reading

L Registrar MRCGP candidates perform relatively poorly in organisational and management questions. They often come across to examiners as reluctant to take responsibility for the non-clinical parts of practice – the parts that will largely govern your future income!

Final phase   The last couple of months of the training year go very quickly. Suddenly the end is nigh and you realise how much more you need to learn and achieve. Your trainer's report should be submitted by the end of month 11. Your VTR/1 form will need to be completed by the trainer and Director of Postgraduate GP Education so that you can apply for your JCPTGP certificate. Also, the MRCGP examination might loom large and decisions about your personal and career plans have to be made. Now more than ever you understand that the registrar year is just a springboard for your future learning and this is a good time to think about how you approach your continuing medical education and professional development.

L In the MRCGP, and particularly in the orals, examiners will be looking to see if you have made active use of your registrar year to begin a lifelong commitment to your ongoing personal and professional growth. They will be impressed if you have cultivated enthusiasm and curiosity, can question assumptions and ask relevant questions, can accept responsibility without having to have your hand held too much, and have your own original thoughts about how things could be done better. They won't let you get away with answers beginning, 'In my training practice what they always do is ...'

Ending relationships with colleagues and patients can be difficult and it is wise to give warning of your imminent departure and discuss how your role might be covered after you leave.

Where to next?

For most of us, once we have made the decision to go into general practice, life – in terms of career planning – has been fairly predictable until this point. At the end of the GP registrar year many different paths open up. Some will move directly into partnership, although this straight transition is much less common than it once was and numerous different jobs or combinations of jobs are possible once you have gained your JCPTGP certificate. For some this uncertainty about the future can be unsettling but try to regard it as a privilege and an opportunity to have a wide variety of options opening up for you.

One recent and welcome development in most areas is the availability, through Deaneries, of a limited number of extended GP training programmes, sometimes known as GP Senior Registrar posts. These posts allow registrars, if selected, to extend their training by 6 months. They combine further supervised general practice experience (usually four sessions per week) with other educational experience in one or more clinical specialties relevant to general practice and/or academic (i.e. research/teaching) experience.

At the end of training, assuming you intend to work as a GP for at least part of your time, you have in broad terms two options. These are to work as a GP Principal or as a non-principal. Principals are basically partners in a practice; the term 'non-principal' covers doctors who work as GP assistants, salaried GPs, GP retainers, locums, GP deputies or for GP cooperatives.

Partnership is traditionally regarded as the ultimate objective of GP training. There are indeed many advantages in terms of continuity, stability, security, having a role in shaping and delivering a service and becoming part of a community. There is also usually financial advantage compared with working as a non-principal. The perceived disadvantages are that although it is no longer assumed that a partnership is necessarily for life, at least a medium-term (say 5 years) commitment is usually expected. There are also greater responsibilities to bear in terms of ongoing patient care, providing out-of-hours cover, employing staff and managing finance and premises.

Many registrars do not feel ready to step straight into partnership after qualification. They might not be sure of whereabouts they wish to settle or which sort of practice they want to work in long term. This is a good time to work flexibly as a non-principal and sample different sorts of working environments, all the time building upon your clinical experience. Some doctors might also choose to combine part-time general practice with other work, for example, in hospital or non-GP community posts, teaching, research or writing. Others might take a complete break to work outside medicine, travel or start a family. Useful guidance on the opportunities and requirements of working as a non-principal can be sought from the National Association of Non-Principals, whose website is www.nanp.org.uk.

The landscape of general practice is changing (see Chapter 16) and the principal/non-principal divide might look quite different in years to come. In the meantime, although flexibility and variety are stimulating for a time, most of us will eventually be drawn to the security and satisfaction of working, at least part-time, in one practice with the stable group of patients and colleagues that partnership provides.

Summary

- The move from working as a hospital doctor into general practice is both daunting and exciting. To get the most out of it you should take care to choose a practice and trainer suited to your needs.

- As well as making sure you understand the formal training and assessment requirements, take time to consider your own personal aims for the registrar year and discuss with your trainer early on how you will approach achieving these aims.

- Be aware of the 'phases' involved in the year and make sure you plan, at the start, a calendar for the year to include all your learning objectives and summative assessment deadlines. Your plan should include thinking – before the very end – about your next career move after completing the registrar year.

- Make the most of all the learning opportunities that come your way, be they related to your trainer, other members of the practice or local services, peers in your half-day release group and, most of all, your patients.

References

Department of Health 2000 The GP registrar scheme, vocational training for general medical practice, the UK guide. Online. Available: www.doh.gov.uk/medicaltraingintheuk

Department of Health and Welsh Office 2002 NHS general medical services statement of fees and allowances. HMSO, London. Online. Available: www.nhs.uk/redbook/

Neighbour R 1992 The inner apprentice. Kluwer Academic, Dordrecht

Pereira Gray D 1977 A system of training for general practitioners. RCGP Occasional paper 4. RCGP, London

Further reading

Abrams W, Howell S 2002 The GP registrar survival guide. BIOS Scientific Publishers Ltd, Oxford

Chambers R, Mohanna K, Field S 2000 Options and opportunities in medical careers. Radcliffe Medical Press, Abingdon, Oxfordshire

Field S 2000 Vocational training for general practice, career focus. British Medical Journal 321:S2

GMC Tomorrow's Doctors. Recommendations on undergraduate medical education 1993. GMC, London

JCPTGP 2001 A guide to certification. Online. Available: www.jcptgp.org.uk

O'Connell S (ed) 1998 Handbook for non-principals in general practice. NANP Limited Edition Press, Chichester. Online. Available: www.nanp.org.uk

Useful contacts

Royal College of General Practitioners
Information sheets available via www.rcgp.org.uk/rcgp/information

2 Summative assessment of GP training

Joe Rosenthal

In the context of education, assessment is whatever is done to measure or judge the progress of learning. Assessment can take many forms; some activities are done by the learners themselves (self-assessment), some by teachers and some by institutions – schools/colleges or professional examining bodies.

Educationalists make a distinction between two main types of assessment, which they call *formative* assessment and *summative* assessment: Formative assessment is the monitoring and testing of progress that goes on during any course or learning process and that helps to inform and shape the educational process. Summative assessment is an 'end-point assessment', that is, usually some form of objective test or examination taking place at the end of a period of education or training, which sums up what has been learned by that point in time. An example of formative assessment is an end-of-firm long case examination at medical school, which does not count towards finals or affect progression; an example of a summative assessment is an end-of-year exam that must be passed to progress onto the next year of the course. Formative assessment might be said to exist primarily for the learner; summative assessment might be said to exist primarily for the learning institution. As you will realise, the distinction is not entirely black and white and, ideally, summative assessment is also formative in that it ends only one period of learning in an ongoing process and thereby informs the shape of future learning.

Summative assessment in GP training

Since 1996, the Joint Committee on Postgraduate Training in General Practice (JCPTGP) and Regional Advisers in General Practice have been committed to having an objective test of all GP registrars' skills, ensuring that those completing training achieve a minimum level of competence to practise independently as general practitioners in the NHS. This objective test is called summative assessment (SA) and the NHS (Vocational Training for General Medical Practice) Regulations 1997 made the passing of summative assessment mandatory by law for all doctors who started their GP registrar post after 30 January 1998. Since that time, to gain accreditation and start practising as a GP in the UK, whether as a principal, assistant, salaried GP or locum, a doctor must have passed summative assessment.

Summative assessment is designed to be a test of minimum competence (unlike MRCGP, which is test of excellence; see Chapter 3) in the wide range of knowledge, skills and attitudes required for an independent practitioner in general medical practice. The pass standard is set at a constant level so there is no built-in failure rate and the intention is that the vast majority of GP registrars who complete their training both in hospital and in their general practice attachment should have no difficulty in passing this assessment.

> **L** The MRCGP exam is also primarily a summative assessment. This is not always appreciated by failing candidates, who often ask for detailed analysis of the reasons for their failure in order to prepare to retake it. Formative feedback on all the exam's modules is limited to statistical and computer-held information.

Assessment has always formed an important part of the GP training process, even before summative assessment became a formal requirement. At the start of training, registrars usually complete an initial assessment to confirm their current level of knowledge. This may be informal by discussion and observation or more formally using MCQs (multiple choice questions) or MEQs (modified essay questions), for example. Formative assessment to determine whether sufficient progress is being made continues throughout the training, again both through case discussion and observation and with the help of assessment tools such as MCQs, MEQs, presentations, video and observed consultations. Thus, until 1996 assessment of GP trainees was largely formative, with assessment methods and policies varying between different Regions and trainers. The only requirements to proceed from vocational training were signed certificates of satisfactory completion of the appropriate 2 years' hospital posts and the year as a trainee/registrar in a training practice. The MRCGP examination has been available since 1965 and was taken by many trainees, but it has never been a requirement for continuing in practice.

L It is often said that 'assessment drives learning', i.e. the content of an examination steers the educational focus of candidates and their teachers. With an eye to spotting potential exam topics, ask yourself what aspects of practice might currently be considered 'weak spots' that the College might like to see registrars giving more attention to.

In the early 1990s there was enormous debate about the wisdom of the introduction of summative assessment, with many trainers and course organisers feeling that the existing system was quite appropriate for adult learners in a vocational setting. There was concern that the imposition of a rigid end-point assessment was a regressive educational step and that trainees would be forced to focus their learning during the year on those measurable elements used in summative assessment at the expense of time spent developing their skills in the many aspects of general practice, which are more qualitative and difficult to assess in any formal way. There was also little evidence that the current system was producing poor-quality GPs or that introducing summative assessment would improve quality. Political and general professional pressure, however, was strongly in favour of objective assessment and so the proponents of summative assessment won the day.

L The political context of summative assessment (and the regulatory framework of GP performance in general) is a fertile ground for MRCGP questions, especially in the orals. You might well be asked about the merits and demerits of the existing system or proposed changes to it. There are no 'right' or 'wrong' opinions but the examiners would expect you to have rational, well-informed and defensible views.

In spite of their reservations and objections, most GP educators accept that summative assessment does have a number of important benefits:

■ It ensures that patients are provided with the protection of knowing that all doctors who complete general practice vocational training will have had their competence assessed to a national standard.
■ It reassures individual doctors that they have achieved an agreed minimum standard of competence.

- It identifies those who are not ready for independent practice and who require further training or who need to reconsider their career options.
- It removes the responsibility from trainers of being the sole assessor of competence.

The organisation of summative assessment

The National Summative Assessment Board is responsible for administering, monitoring and, in some cases, organising, the provision of methods of summative assessment. The Board is an umbrella body for the delivery of all methods of summative assessment in the UK. It operates on behalf of the Conference of General Practice Education Directors (COGPED) with the purpose of supervising the administration of the various methods of summative assessment, approved by the JCPTGP, in the Deaneries. The work of the Board and its Chair is supported by the National Office for Summative Assessment, based at King Alfred's College, Winchester (useful information is available on its website: www.doctoronline.nhs.uk). Each Deanery has a Summative Assessment Office, which administers the COGPED component parts of summative assessment, that is, the video of consulting skills, audit, MCQ, structured trainer's report and the MRCGP/SA single-route video (see below). To ensure national consistency and reliability in the programme and marking of submissions, the Deanery Offices are bound by a protocol agreement approved by the JCPTGP and are required to submit a random selection of audits and videos for quality control to the national panel for summative assessment. At the start of your registrar year, you should receive a detailed summative assessment pack from your Deanery, which will also have up-to-date information on its website.

What does summative assessment involve?

Summative assessment is now well established but still evolving (Box 2.1). The general information given here was up-to-date at the time of writing but it is likely that changes will occur over time. It is worth checking the official national guidance (which can be downloaded in full from www.doctoronline.nhs.uk together with application forms, marking schedules and the structured trainer's report form). You should also make sure you are fully informed of any local variations in your own area by seeking up-to-date information from your Regional Deanery. Deanery Offices will issue a summative assessment guide and number to all their GP registrars at the beginning of their registrarship. You should ensure that you know your number and that it appears on all your submissions and correspondence.

L The regulations governing summative assessment specify the areas of competence to be assessed but not the standard required. Why do you think this is? What are the difficulties in deciding what constitutes 'minimum competence'? Who should be involved in setting this standard?

Box 2.1
What does summative assessment assess?

> According to the regulations, the competencies tested by summative assessment are:
>
> 1 Factual medical knowledge, which is sufficient to enable the practitioner to perform the duties of a general practitioner.
> 2 The ability to apply factual medical knowledge to the management of problems presented by patients in general practice.
> 3 Effective communication, both orally and in writing.
> 4 The ability to consult satisfactorily with general practice patients.
> 5 The ability to review and critically analyse the practitioner's own working practices and manage any necessary changes appropriately.
> 6 Clinical skills.
> 7 The ability to synthesise all the above competencies and apply them appropriately in a general practice setting.

At present, the summative assessment test consists of four modules:

- multiple choice questionnaire (MCQ)
- written submission of practical work (e.g. a clinical audit or project under the National Project Marking Schedule; see p. 22)
- assessment of consultation skills, using video or simulated surgery (e.g. the Leicester/Yorkshire Simulated Patient Surgery)
- structured trainer's report.

All four modules must be passed to complete summative assessment successfully. The procedure for each module and instructions for candidates are given in the booklet *Summative Assessment General Practice Training*, published by the Conference of Postgraduate Advisers in General Practice Universities of the United Kingdom. All GP registrars should receive an information pack and a copy of the booklet from their Dean of Postgraduate General Practice Education.

Once all four components have been successfully completed, your trainer will sign a VTR1 form. This, together with the VTR2 forms from your hospital jobs, should be sent to the office of the Dean of Postgraduate General Practice Education for your Region where they will be checked, endorsed and forwarded to the Joint Committee on Postgraduate Training in General Practice (JCPTGP), who in turn will issue a Statement of Satisfactory Completion.

The MCQ   There are two options for the MCQ examination. One is to take the exam set by the UK Conference of Regional Advisers (UKCRA) and the other is to sit the MRCGP MCQ exam. The UKCRA examination tests knowledge and problem-solving skills and is set at the level of medical school finals. It is held four times each year at several venues around the UK. There are around 300 machine-marked items of true or false questions and extended matching questions for which you are allowed 3 hours. There is no negative marking. The pass rate is currently around 94% but, should you fail, you can re-sit the exam on up to two further occasions. The questions cover the full range of activities that are part of modern general practice. GP registrars are advised that they can take the assessment after completing 3 months in general practice and when they and their trainers agree they are ready.

An increasingly popular alternative to the UKCRA MCQ examination is to sit the MCQ paper of the MRCGP examination, a pass in which automatically exempts you from the summative assessment MCQ. More details on this are given in Chapter 3.

The written submission of practical work

The written submission is a test of the ability to:

1 construct a logical argument and communicate it in written English
2 plan and sustain activity over time.

The written submission is commonly referred to as 'the audit', because this is the type of submission chosen by most registrars. A completed audit cycle – including the implementation of change and a second collection of data – is the favoured method in many Deaneries (see Chapter 10 for more on audit). Remember, the golden rule here is to keep it simple and avoid being overambitious. A small, well-focused and relevant audit (Box 2.2) will take less time to prepare and is more likely to bring about change. A lot of very useful guidance on preparing an audit is available on websites such as that provided by Dr John Schofield for the London Deanery, at www.londondeanery.ac.uk/gp/home.htm.

As an alternative to an audit, you can submit a variety of written projects under the National Project Marking Schedule (NPMS), which has been approved by the JCPTGP since April 2000. A project is defined as a self-directed piece of learning that:

- addresses a defined problem
- is related to previous work
- presents qualitative or quantitative findings

Box 2.2
Recommended headings for audit report

- Title
- Reason for choice of audit
- Audit criteria chosen
- Standards set
- Preparation and planning
- First data collection
- Changes to be evaluated
- Second data collection
- Conclusions – summary of main issues learned

More details are available from the National Office for Summative Assessment via www.doctoronline.nhs.uk

- interprets these findings
- draws conclusions from the evidence presented.

Examples of the sorts of submission to NPMS include:

- a simple research study
- an audit of any type
- a literature review
- a case study
- a proposal for a new service in the practice
- a discussion paper.

The NPMS describes each level of achievement so that registrars are clear as to what is required. Full details of NPMS are available from the Yorkshire Deanery (see the Useful contacts section at the end of this chapter).

The assessment of consulting skills

There are currently three approved assessments of consulting skills:

1 submit a video for summative assessment purposes only
2 submit a video for the consulting skills module of the MRCGP examination
3 apply to have your skills tested by a simulated patient surgery.

A detailed discussion of learning and assessing consultation skills appears in Chapter 4. Always check up-to-date advice from your Deanery but, at the time of writing, the video required for summative assessment should be recorded on VHS 'standard play' and contain 2 h of (a minimum of eight) consultations. The tape should demonstrate your performance at a varied level of challenge. An accompanying log book provides a chance to explain the circumstances of the consultation and what you were doing. You are not asked to submit a masterpiece but the consultation must be free from major errors that might put a patient at risk, or collections of minor errors that might cause inconvenience or embarrassment.

An alternative and potentially more challenging and satisfying video assessment is the consulting skills module of the MRCGP examination. Again the bare bones of an effective consultation are covered but you will also be required to demonstrate a patient-centred consulting style. Like the MCQ, a pass in the MRCGP video module gains exemption from summative assessment. Should you not be successful, your videotape will be automatically 'fast-tracked' through local summative assessment procedures. Over 90% of candidates who fail the MRCGP video will go on to pass summative assessment.

Details of the simulated patient surgeries held in the Yorkshire Deanery (for candidates in the northern half of the UK) and Trent Deanery (for candidates in the southern half of the UK) are to be found in the national guidance. They are held in spring and autumn and each surgery involves eight consultations and lasts about 2½ h. Actors play patients and you are allowed 5 min between patients to complete a postencounter form and

Box 2.3
*The six sections of
the structured
trainer's report*

1 Patient care (divided into general clinical skills, patient
   management skills and clinical judgement)
2 Communication skills
3 Personal and professional growth
4 Organisational skills
5 Professional values
6 Specific clinical skills (divided into diagnostic skills and
   emergency care)

clinical checklist. You must pass six consultations or you will be asked
to repeat. If you fail the repeat surgery you will be referred to an expert
panel. Familiarisation sessions are arranged twice a year and you should
contact your Deanery for further details (see the Useful contacts section
at the end of this chapter).

The structured trainer's report

The trainer's report is a comprehensive summary of your clinical and
organisational skills, your ability to diagnose and manage patients, and
an assessment of your professional values and personal and professional growth (Box 2.3). Trainers should point out identified weaknesses during your training period, allowing time and plenty of support
to work on those areas that you might find more difficult.

The report form gives guidance to the trainers on the minimum standards – what will constitute a pass or fail – and registrars are well advised
to read a blank report form early on in the year to see what criteria they
are judged on and to discuss these with their trainer at regular intervals.

Most of the trainer's report will be completed at the beginning of the
last 2 months of training.

Trainers are also given guidance as to the best method of assessment
under three categories: assessment by observation, assessment by discussion and assessment by specific methods.

All items will need to be completed satisfactorily for the trainer's
report to be submitted, 2 months before the completion of training.
Trainers have been instructed that whenever there is any doubt about
whether or not the GP registrar has reached the necessary standard,
repeat observation should be made. Clearly, a trainer who is aware that
a GP registrar is as yet unable to reach the required standard will
arrange for appropriate training and seek the advice of a course organiser, associate adviser or regional adviser.

Planning for summative assessment

A full and detailed description of the requirements and process of summative assessment will be sent to you from your Deanery at the beginning
of your registrar year, together with your national summative assessment
number. Take some time to read through the national guidance with your
trainer and decide which of the various methods of assessment you
wish to opt for. Having done this, complete your summative assessment

Table 2.1
Summative Assessment Planner

Month	Action
Month 1	Read the summative assessment guidance that has been sent to you by your Deanery. Also read the National Trainer's Report form so that you know what will be expected of you by the end of the year. Discuss your summative assessment plans with your trainer
Month 2	Check when and where the next MCQ is being held Consider a topic for written submission Practise video-recording consultations
Months 3–4	Complete and return the summative assessment application form Start collecting data if doing an audit for your written submission Start keeping videos for the video submission
Month 5	You should be well on the way to completing your video and audit. If confident, attempt the MCQ this month
Months 6–7	The video and audit should be submitted between now and month 9. Don't leave it too late because you will need time to resubmit if you don't pass first time If planning to sit the MRCGP examination, apply by the end of month 6
Month 8	The deadline for submitting the single route MRCGP/SA video is this month. Simulated surgeries are held between months 8 and 10
Month 9	The deadline for the video and audit is the end of this month
Months 10–11	Your trainer should submit the trainer's report by the end of month 11, together with a signed VTR1
Month 12	JCPTGP issues a Statement of Satisfactory Completion

application form and return it to your Deanery. Form a year plan, based on Table 2.1, to help you keep to the required summative assessment timetable.

Getting your results

Your results will be sent out by the Deanery Summative Assessment Administrator by letter; they are not given over the telephone. You can expect to receive them as follows:

1 MCQ – at least 3 weeks after the examination
2 Audit – 5 weeks after receipt by Deanery
3 Video – 8 weeks after receipt by Deanery.

There are three possible outcomes: pass, referral or fail. If you are unhappy with the way your summative assessment submissions were processed, there is an appeals procedure, a copy of which can be obtained from the Deanery Summative Assessment Administrator. If you think, that you have underperformed for some other reason (e.g. illness, transport delays), you can lodge an appeal with the Deanery, but only before results have been made available.

If you do not pass

If a particular component of the summative assessment other than the MCQ (i.e. the written submission, video or trainer's report) is considered borderline or poor it will be referred to a second or third level of assessment.

For the written submission, if a pass is still not deemed appropriate after referral the work is returned for resubmission after further specific training. For the video, should a pass not be obtained after referral, GP registrars will be asked to submit another video-tape after further specific training. This tape should not normally be submitted less than 6 months from the date of the first submission. Under exceptional circumstances this may be earlier if the Regional Deanery believes this to be desirable. In the event that this specific period of video training cannot be completed within the normal duration of vocational training, then the GP registrar will need to seek an extension of his or her training. In the event of failure of the second video submission, the Regional Deanery will discuss the matter and how to proceed with the GP registrar and others involved in his or her training.

A borderline or poor trainer's report will be referred to consultation with course organisers or associate advisers, who will recommend what action needs to be taken. Ultimate failure of the overall summative assessment is likely to be rare because it is a test of minimum competence. However, in the unlikely event of failure, additional training time within the Deanery – usually up to a maximum of 6 months – can usually be made available. If you are having problems along the way, discuss them as soon as possible with your trainer and course organiser.

Summary

- Passing summative assessment is an essential requirement to gain accreditation to practise independently as a GP in the UK.

- Summative assessment is designed as a test of minimum competence and the expectation is that the vast majority of registrars will pass without difficulty.

- The four elements of summative assessment are the MCQ, assessment of consultation skills, the written submission and the structured trainer's report. You must include completing all these elements in your Registrar year plan, but take care not to let these hoops and hurdles dominate your year at the expense of the many other formative learning opportunities that will come your way.

- Ensure you are clear about the national and local summative assessment requirements, which you should receive in a summative assessment pack from your postgraduate Deanery.

- Remember also to consider the MRCGP/SA single route. This allows you to submit the same consultation video and/or sit the same MCQ examination to satisfy both assessments.

Acknowledgements

We are very grateful to Dr Tim Swanwick of London Deanery for detailed information from the London Deanery SA web pages, which you can see at www.londondeanery.ac.uk/gp/home.htm

Further reading

Abrams W, Howell S 2002 The GP registrar survival guide. BIOS Scientific Publishers, Oxford

Committee of General Practice Education Directors 2001 Summative assessment for general practice. Online. Available: www.doctoronline.nhs.uk

London Deanery Summative Assessment Guide. Online. Available: www.londondeanery.ac.uk/home.htm

Useful contacts

Trent Deanery (for candidates in the southern UK)
Tel: 0116 253 8118

Yorkshire Deanery (for candidates in the northern UK)
Tel: 01434 554448

3 The MRCGP examination

Roger Neighbour

Passing summative assessment at the end of your registrar year shows that you have at least 'a minimum level of competence to practise independently' as a GP (Vocational Training Summative Assessment Board 1998). In other words, the standard is set at a level just high enough to ensure that you are not positively dangerous. It puts you in approximately the top 97% of your peers – not anything to be particularly proud of, and indeed, most people would agree that patients ought to expect a considerably higher standard from their doctors. The MRCGP represents that higher standard. At the moment, approximately 90% of registrars take the examination and about 80% of those will pass at their first or second attempt. This chapter explains why you might want to aspire to the MRCGP, what is involved in reaching it and how you might set about achieving this goal.

Why take the MRCGP?

In its constitution, the Royal College of General Practitioners (RCGP) states its object as being 'to encourage, foster and maintain the highest possible standards in general medical practice ...'. At the bottom of every sheet of RCGP headed paper is its mission statement: 'Promoting excellence in family medicine'. Whether or not you like this sort of thing, I hope that, after anything up to 10 years of study and preparation, you would want finish your training knowing that you are as good as you *can* be, and not merely as good as you *need* to be.

The RCGP has deliberately set the content and standard of its Membership examination to be appropriate to the end-point of vocational training. It allows for the fact that, whereas your level of theoretical knowledge is probably quite high, some of the skills and competences that only come with experience will not yet be fully developed. In fact, some doctors who delay taking the exam until later in their career find its written elements quite taxing, because they have got out of the habit of keeping on top of general practice's constantly evolving knowledge base. On the other hand, the standard expected in the exam's oral and consulting skills components is well within the reach of any registrar who has made the most of the training year's opportunities to explore some of the 'softer' and more subtle dimensions of practice.

This being the case, if you successfully measure your competence against the College's Membership requirements, you will have achieved an accolade you can be justly proud of. Having MRCGP after your name is evidence of your own values. It shows you have set yourself a high standard to live up to and that your patients can expect to receive competent, up-to-date, compassionate and patient-centred care.

At the time of writing, the MRCGP is a voluntary qualification rather than a mandatory one. That is to say that, unlike the equivalent qualifications for physicians and surgeons (MRCP, FRCS), it is not an absolute requirement for going into practice. However, this may change within the next few years. The College is committed to promoting MRCGP as the sine qua non for becoming a principal in general practice, and some Health Authorities already have such a policy in place. Moreover, it is highly likely that, as professional revalidation becomes established, there will be some form of linkage with College membership. If at some future stage in your career you wish to become a trainer or course organiser, you will find that virtually every Region will expect you to have attained the MRCGP.

If I can suggest it without sounding too pompous, you might also consider there is a professional responsibility to align yourself with an institution that stands for high academic standards in general practice. The history of our discipline is of a struggle to define and promote the unique virtues of 'the specialty of generalism'. The RCGP has worked for half a century to establish itself as the focus for all that is precious about personal doctoring. The more GPs who are willing to nail their own colours to the College's mast, the greater the chance that future generations of patients will benefit from this tradition.

> **L** The MRCGP is currently a voluntary qualification. Have you decided to take the exam? If not, what will be the implications if it becomes mandatory if you want to work for a Health Authority that has a policy of employing only Members of the RCGP as principals?

A brief history

The College of General Practitioners was founded in 1953 and received its Royal Charter in 1967. In its early years, membership was solely upon application, but in 1965 an entry examination was introduced. Five candidates sat, and all passed. Since then, numbers of candidates have climbed steadily, reaching a peak of over 2000 in 1998. When summative assessment came on-stream there was a temporary dip in applications for the exam, probably because registrars felt the additional workload was a distraction from the essential but time-consuming task of demonstrating minimum competence. However, as registrars have found this need not be the case, and as some parts of the MRCGP examination have secured exemption from summative assessment, candidate numbers have recovered. Currently, about 1800 UK registrars enter for the MRCGP exam each year, and this number is expected to climb still further.

Until the mid-1980s the examination consisted of a multiple choice question (MCQ) testing factual knowledge, a modified essay question (MEQ) testing the application of knowledge, a practice topic or essay question (PTQ) and two orals, one based on the candidate's own clinical diary. In 1985, the Chief Examiner at the time lamented in print the apparent reluctance of candidates to read published literature. The heated debate that followed led to the replacement of the PTQ by a critical reading question (CRQ), testing candidates' ability to interpret and apply contemporary research literature.

In 1997, after nearly a decade of development, a test of consulting skills was introduced. For most candidates, this involves submitting a video-tape of selected consultations: Chapter 4 addresses this topic in more detail. Candidates having insuperable difficulty in providing a video-tape can have their consulting skills assessed by a simulated surgery in which they consult with role-playing patients. Registrar readers of this book are, however, unlikely to be eligible for this alternative during their training year.

The MRCGP used to be an 'all or none' exam. All elements had to be sat at the same time and failure in any one part meant failure overall: if you failed one part you could not carry over successes in another part when resitting the component you had failed. This seemed to place arbitrary and unnecessary constraints on the exam's appeal to busy registrars and, in 1998, the MRCGP changed to a modular format. Details are given below, but essentially each component of the exam can now be taken separately over a 3-year period, and successes accumulated until all have been passed. This format has proved extremely popular with candidates. One consequence has been that each module must now have 'stand alone' reliability and, as a result, the content of the former CRQ has been subsumed within the MCQ and a restructured written paper. The orals too have been streamlined, and now consist of two 20-min orals focusing mainly on decision-making and professional values.

In recent years, the MRCGP exam has been criticised for its frequent changes in structure. As someone largely responsible for this, however, I make no apology. General practice itself is in a period of rapid change and our notions of what forms of assessment are relevant, fair and feasible have had to keep pace with it. I hope you will be reassured by the knowledge that the MRCGP now leads the world as an assessment of primary care, in terms of both its academic credentials and its reputation for helpfulness to candidates.

The exam's structure and content

Before describing the MRCGP's structure and content in detail, let us say this: *Full and up-to-date details are available, and **only** available, from the Examination Department at the RCGP. The Regulations are updated annually and you could be seriously misled if you do not refer to the current version* (see the Useful contacts section at the end of this chapter). Although the information in these pages is correct at the time of going to press, you should not rely on this or any other book as a source of accurate information about the rules and procedures in force at the time you sit the examination. Always contact the Examination Department for guidance. Having largely written them, I know that the Examination Regulations are a comprehensive and reliable guide to how the exam is conducted!

> **L** Have you made a note of the contact details of the RCGP Examination Department? You will need to contact them to receive the up-to-date Examination Regulations, which are a reliable guide to how the exam will be conducted.

Structure

The MRCGP is a credit accumulation examination. This means that:

- you must pass all four modules of the exam to pass overall
- the modules can be taken at the same session or in different sessions, in any order
- you can, on payment of the appropriate fee, have up to two further attempts at each module
- all modules must be passed within 3 years of your application being accepted, otherwise you must retake the whole examination.

The four modules are:

- a written paper
- a multiple choice paper
- an assessment of consulting skills
- an oral examination.

Each module is available twice a year, in the summer and the winter.

You must also provide evidence of proficiency in basic cardiopulmonary resuscitation and child health surveillance. Details will be provided when you apply to take the exam.

The written paper

The written paper lasts 3½ h, including time allowed for reading any articles or material on which questions are based. It consists of 12 questions, which are to be answered in prose or short notes format. There are typically four question types:

1 Questions designed to test your knowledge and interpretation of general practice literature. You are expected to be familiar with significant items in the medical literature that impinge on current or important issues in general practice.
2 Questions that test your ability to evaluate and interpret written material presented to you (e.g. excerpts from published papers).
3 Questions that examine your ability to integrate and apply theoretical knowledge and professional values.
4 New question formats: the examiners reserve the right to ask questions on topics, or in formats, that test your responsiveness to the changing face of primary care.

The multiple choice paper

Unlike the written paper, which is hand-marked by examiners, the multiple choice paper is computer-marked by an Opscan machine. You indicate your answers by filling in lozenges on the answer sheet, which is supplied at the time of the examination. This paper is designed to test both your knowledge of the theoretical base of general practice and, more importantly, the deeper understanding and application of that knowledge. The paper lasts 3 h and contains up to 250 separate items. The questions examine:

- core knowledge
- emerging knowledge (i.e. recent advances)

- application of knowledge
- critical appraisal, including statistics and research methodology.

There are a number of different question formats:

- extended matching questions, in which a scenario has to be matched to an answer from a list of options
- single best-answer questions, in which a statement or stem is followed by a variable number of items, only one of which is correct
- multiple best-answer questions, in which a statement is followed by a variable number of items, a specified number of which might be correct
- summary completion questions, which test your critical reading ability from a summary of a paper presented in the question paper
- multiple true/false questions, which comprise a statement followed by a number of items, any or all or none of which might be correct.

The consulting skills component

Your consulting skills are assessed by one of two methods:

1 you submit video recordings of yourself consulting with real patients in your own surgery
2 you take part in a 'simulated surgery', in which you consult with a series of standardised patients who are portrayed by role-players.

The video recording is the MRCGP's normal method and most registrar candidates working in training practices will go down this route. The video method is described Chapter 4.

The simulated surgery option is only available to candidates who can make a case for having insuperable difficulties in producing a suitable video, for example if you are no longer working in general practice or if most of your consultations are not conducted in English. If you think you might be eligible for the simulated surgery option, you should follow the procedures set out in the Exam Regulations. Full details would be sent to you once your application had been approved.

In the simulated surgery, you are stationed in a room arranged to resemble a consulting room. A series of role-play 'patients' (currently 12, although the number could vary) consult you at 10-min intervals, as if you were conducting a routine surgery. The role-players undergo extensive training and rehearsal to make sure they can reproduce the same presentation to a variety of doctors, and are extremely realistic. They present problems designed to allow you to demonstrate your communication and consulting skills. Each 'patient' is accompanied by an examiner, who silently observes and marks the consultation.

The orals

The oral component consists of two 20-min orals, each with two examiners. The orals aim to assess your communication skills, your professional values and your personal and professional growth in the contexts of:

- the care of individual patients
- working with colleagues

- the social role of general practice
- your personal responsibilities.

Each oral covers approximately five topics. You are not required to bring details of any of your own cases.

Content

The discipline of general practice has few fixed boundaries, being defined as much by what patients elect to present to us as by our own views on the GP's job description. General practice is constantly evolving, reflecting advances in clinical practice, shifts in social expectations and changes in the political, administrative and fiscal framework. There is therefore no fixed syllabus for the MRCGP. It sets out to test all those areas of professional knowledge, skills and values that reflect the consensus view of what constitutes good practice in the UK NHS.

The Panel of Examiners is guided by the following blueprint, which describes in general terms the domains of competence required of a contemporary GP:

- factual knowledge
- evolving knowledge: 'hot topics', qualitative research
- the evidence base of practice; knowledge of literature, quantitative research
- critical appraisal skills: interpretation of literature, principles of statistics
- application of knowledge: justification, prioritising, audit
- problem-solving: clinical management, decision-making
- personal care: matching principles to individual patients
- written communication
- verbal communication: the consultation process
- the practice context: team issues, practice management, business skills
- the regulatory framework of practice
- the wider context: medico-political, legal and societal issues
- ethnic and transcultural issues
- values and attitudes: ethics, integrity, consistency
- self-awareness: insight, 'the doctor as a person'
- maintaining standards: personal and professional growth, continuing medical education.

Within each module, a variety of contexts is examined to test an appropriate range and depth. You might find it helpful to consider all the various roles the GP might adopt in the course of everyday practice, for example:

- clinician
- family physician
- patient's advocate
- gatekeeper
- resource allocator

- handler of information
- team member
- team leader
- partner
- colleague
- employer
- manager
- business-person
- learner
- teacher
- reflective practitioner
- researcher
- agent and shaper of policy
- member of a profession
- spouse and/or parent
- person and individual.

The 'philosophy' of the MRCGP exam

The MRCGP enjoys, and jealously guards, a reputation as one of the most highly regarded postgraduate exams in primary care in the world. Indeed, it forms the template for equivalent examinations in an increasing number of countries – worldwide – who are developing their own local examinations, which, if they can demonstrate parity with the MRCGP for rigour and standard, will be awarded 'MRCGP International' status.

Setting the standard required to pass any exam is essentially a philosophical decision rather than a purely numerical or academic one. It reflects the parent organisation's compromise between what is desirable and what is fair and feasible. The MRCGP aims to set a standard that reflects credit on the successful candidate and in which patients can have confidence. There is no intrinsically logical reason for a pass mark to be set at 50% (or any other predetermined percentage, for that matter). Neither, unless the exam is acting as a 'turnstile' to allow only a fixed number of candidates through in order to control access to subsequent career stages, is there any reason for it to pass any preset proportion of the candidates who sit it. The MRCGP currently has an overall pass rate of the order of 75–80%. (An exact figure is hard to establish in a modular exam allowing multiple re-sits.) A pass rate of this order is felt to have the most constructive effect on the motivation and learning behaviour of potential candidates. It is low enough to carry a real danger of failure if the necessary preparation is not undertaken but not so low as to discourage the majority of registrar candidates from attempting something well within their reach.

A catch-phrase in education is that 'assessment drives learning': if candidates expect to be examined on certain topics, they prepare for them. From the examiners' point of view, an effective way of sending educational messages to the vocational training establishment is to raise the exam profile of aspects of practice that are felt to need greater attention. The MRCGP exam does this quite unashamedly. The example of the introduction of a critical reading element has already been given. The advent of the consulting skills component signalled the RCGP's belief that patient-centred consulting skills are central to good practice, and the beneficial effect on candidates' consulting style is now becoming clear. Others examples in recent years include curriculum-setting questions on alcohol problems, family dynamics and the non-journal literature of general practice.

The MRCGP is a 'criterion-referenced' or 'norm-referenced' exam, rather than a peer-referenced one. This means that, in deciding whether a particular candidate passes or fails, he or she is assessed against a fixed objective criterion or norm rather than his or her performance being compared against that of the other candidates. Norm referencing, which theoretically means that 100% of candidates could pass if they all met the criteria, is generally considered the fairer option. For the examiners it is not the easier option, however. Much work goes into clarifying and defining the criteria required to pass and into determining the pass mark on every part and sitting of the exam. Further details of how this is done in the various modules of the exam can be found in the Examination Regulations supplied to candidates, and in the College's own book on the examination (Moore 2000).

When the MRCGP was reconfigured into its present modular format, concern was expressed that some candidates might aim no higher than a bare pass put together module-by-module over a lengthy period of time, and that this might 'devalue the currency'. To offset any such effect, the concept of a 'pass with merit' was introduced. Approximately the top 25% of candidates in each module are awarded a pass with merit. Candidates who obtain a pass with merit in two modules and pass the other two are awarded MRCGP with Merit. Candidates who at their first attempt pass with merit in all four modules, or in three with a pass in the other one, are awarded MRCGP with Distinction.

Reliability

From a candidate's point of view it is always tempting to denigrate any examination − criticism of the assessment method is one of our usual defences against the possibility of being judged unfavourably. Perhaps the exam doesn't look at the relevant skills and topics, or ask pertinent questions, or have sensible marking schedules. Maybe the examiners aren't consistent, so that the result depends too much on which particular examiners the candidate encounters. Perhaps the pass mark is set at the wrong level. From the point of view of an examiner wishing to secure the trust of our candidates, I agree with every one of these concerns. To address them, the MRCGP draws heavily on international expertise in the fields of assessment methodology, and invests significant amounts of time and resources in a rolling programme of quality control.

Any examination is a process of sampling and of generalising. Probably the best way for me to decide if you were a good GP would be to spend several days or weeks watching you at work, and even then we could argue about what 'good' means, or whether my opinion was worth having. Life being too short for this, an exam takes representative samples – biopsies, if you like – of all the possible knowledge, skills, values and competences that are thought necessary, makes a judgement about them, then tries to extrapolate from that judgement, made on only a partial sample, and come to a decision about what picture of the candidate would have emerged had more or different samples been taken. Deciding which and how many samples to take, and what reliance to place on the results, is the province of a branch of statistics called generalisability theory, which has far-reaching implications for the way the MRCGP exam is conducted.

If you take 1000 candidates and administer some test of their ability, the test will 'discriminate' between them, that is, it will identify who performed the worst and who the best, and arrange all the others in rank order in between. The apparent differences between the candidates – the 'variance' – can come about for three reasons. 'Candidate variance' represents the true differences in ability amongst the cohort of candidates, and is what the test is designed to reveal. 'Marker variance' represents differences of opinion between examiners, who might rate the same performance differently according to whether they are 'hawkish' or 'doveish' in their marking. 'Test variance' arises if the test method is to some extent inherently imprecise.

It is impossible to eradicate marker and test variance completely from any assessment. Together they constitute 'noise' in the system and, in the interests of fairness and accuracy, have to be kept to the absolute minimum by paying good attention to test design and to marking protocols. The scale of distortion arising from non-candidate variance can be estimated statistically and, in the MRCGP, appropriate methodological corrections are introduced before final calculations of candidates' marks are done and pass–fail decisions made In the written paper, individual markers' scores are analysed and adjusted to bring them into line with marks awarded by other examiners marking the same question. In the oral and video components, the four or seven examiners, respectively, who have assessed the candidate meet immediately after the initial marking process to review and, if necessary, adjust their scores to reach a consensus decision that all agree to be correct. To be as generous as possible to borderline candidates without compromising standards, in the written and MCQ papers, and in the simulated surgery, candidates whose scores fall below the pass mark by not more than 1 standard error of measurement are deemed to have passed.

The 'reliability' of a test refers to the likelihood that a candidate would get the same result if the test had been sat on another occasion or marked by different examiners. In multi-item tests where all candidates receive the same assessment (e.g. the MCQ and written papers, and the simulated surgery), statistical tests of internal consistency can be performed to gauge the test's reliability. Cronbach's coefficient alpha (technically, an index of split half correlation) is the appropriate statistic. It is a figure between 0 and 1, with a value of 0.80 being generally regarded as acceptable. Those MRCGP modules to which it applies regularly have alphas between 0.85 and 0.90. In modules where the candidates are not all examined on the same material (i.e. the orals and video), other indices of reliability, such as intermarker correlation, factor analysis and 'test–retest' studies are undertaken routinely.

In addition to the statistical monitoring of its performance, the MRCGP has other built-in safeguards to ensure the examiners have consistent standards. The Panel of Examiners is about 150 strong. All are in regular active general practice. References are taken up on potential new examiners, who must then pass the same MCQ sat by candidates. Their core examining skills are scrutinised during a day-long assessment process, following which they have further training in oral and video examining and in marking written scripts. All examiners regularly undergo a video review of their oral examining and receive equal opportunities training. Two external consultants with expertise in assessment theory and psychometrics are contracted to the exam to assist with data analysis and examiner training.

Practicalities

Any doctor eligible to be an independent practitioner of general practice or family medicine, or undergoing vocational training with this in view, is eligible to take the MRCGP examination. If you are already eligible to practise independently, evidence to this effect must be supplied when you apply (e.g. a Certificate of Prescribed or Equivalent Experience issued by the JCPTGP). Overseas candidates must supply the equivalent documentation in an attested English translation. If as a registrar you pass the MRCGP exam before completing vocational training, you may only take up RCGP Membership once you have received and submitted your Certificate of Prescribed or Equivalent Experience.

The written and MCQ papers are available twice a year, usually in May and October. For convenience, they are held on the same day in up to nine centres in the British Isles. They are sometimes available overseas, for example, in Saudi Arabia or Hong Kong, but this should not be assumed. Oral examinations are held in London and Edinburgh approximately 6 weeks after the written papers. Dates of the simulated surgery vary, and would be notified on acceptance of your application. Videos are at present marked twice a year, in May and November. Details of the exact dates of the examination, the closing dates for entries, the arrangements for submitting video tapes and all other details of the examination process are contained in the annually updated Exam Regulations, to which you must refer for accurate information.

The Exam Department will try to help if you have health problems or are affected by special circumstances (e.g. dyslexia, bereavement). You should contact them in writing as far in advance as possible.

The MRCGP and summative assessment

A pass in the MRCGP MCQ paper is recognised by the JCPTGP as conferring exemption from any other test of factual knowledge for the purposes of summative assessment. Likewise, a pass in the MRCGP video component confers exemption from any other summative assessment test of consulting skills.

Since May 2001 it has been possible for registrars sitting both summative assessment and the MRCGP to prepare a single tape acceptable for both purposes. The tape is first marked by the MRCGP examiners, and, if successful, the candidate is also deemed to have passed the summative assessment consulting skills requirement. If the tape is unsuccessful for MRCGP it can, if the candidate has requested it, be passed immediately to the Regional Deaneries and 'fast tracked' through the summative assessment process. In other words, preparing a single tape is a 'can't lose' option for registrars, and has proved extremely popular. Details of the single-track process are supplied by the Exam Department on application.

> **L** Have you considered submitting a single video for the MRCGP video component and the summative assessment process?

Preparing for the MRCGP

A Zen student asked a Master, 'How shall I live a perfect life?' The Master replied, 'First make yourself perfect, then live naturally'.

Something of the same approach is the best way to prepare for the MRCGP exam. Become as good a GP as you can, then take the exam in your stride. One of the myths about the MRCGP is that exam technique and a liberal sprinkling of catchphrases will ensure success. In fact, the examiners are more impressed by someone whose enthusiasm for general practice is genuine, whose concern for patients sincere and for whom learning the craft has been a self-directed adventure. Rather than seeing the exam as yet another mountain to be climbed laboriously, think of it as a not-too-high hurdle over which the natural impetus of a well-spent registrar year should carry you without too much difficulty. Try throughout your registrar year to remain:

- *curious*: cultivate the mind-set of thinking laterally, exploring the ramifications of everyday practice beyond their immediate context
- *committed*: foster the discipline of regular study throughout your training because mastery of your profession requires it, not simply as an exam-centred chore
- *critical*: get into the habit of questioning assumptions, challenging dogma and constantly asking 'Why?' like any 4-year-old.

That said, it would be foolish to go into the exam without having gone to some trouble to make sure you don't have too many blind spots and are able to get your thoughts into the sort of order that will impress the examiners with the breadth and depth of your competence. The commentary boxes throughout the text of this book are designed to help you with this task by alerting you to how the examiner's mind is likely to work.

Learning aids

A bewildering array of educational material is available to MRCGP candidates, much of it excellent but some ill-informed or frankly misleading. What follows is my own (and therefore idiosyncratic) advice: in this, as in all other matters of adult learning, you should evaluate it against your own needs, opinions and experience.

Journals and publications

You should regularly read the *British Medical Journal* and the *British Journal of General Practice*, including – especially – their leading articles and opinion pieces. Pay careful attention to papers dealing with issues of major clinical or medico-political importance, and devise your own method of filing them for revision and discussion purposes. You should also familiarise yourself with circulars and statements put out by the major players in the NHS such as the Department of Health, the National Institute for Clinical Excellence (NICE), the GMC, the RCGP and the BMA. *Clinical Evidence*, the biannual compendium published by the *BMJ*, is of particular value.

Magazines

The general practice 'glossies' usually contain topic-based review articles that are useful summaries of good practice. They also often run series of articles aimed at MRCGP candidates, the quality of which varies. You should take with a pinch of salt anything by an author lacking direct experience with the exam. However, many current examiners contribute to such series and their advice has the merit of coming from a uniquely well-informed source.

Books

Over several generations, British general practice has accumulated its own corpus of 'books of ideas', which continue to influence contemporary practice. Your trainer should help you to identify them. The exam usually contains plenty of opportunity to display your familiarity with this literature.

There are several books aspiring to the status of MRCGP *vade-mecum*. With the exception of the present volume, it is invidious to make specific recommendations, but Keith Palmer's *Notes for the MRCGP* (Palmer 1998) has a deservedly special place in the affections of candidates. (However, examiners have learned to spot a Palmer-quoting candidate a mile off, and take pride in asking questions that elicit first-hand rather than second-hand experience!) As sources of factual knowledge, the

British National Formulary and books in the Oxford 'Pocket' series (e.g. Longmore et al 2001) are exemplary. Radcliffe Medical Press also publishes a list of issue-related titles pitched at the right level of detail (see the Useful contacts section, p. 43).

Videos   Radcliffe Medical Press, in collaboration with the Panel of Examiners, currently produces two video packs to help candidates prepare for the video (Skelton et al 1998) and oral (Gardiner et al 2001) components of the MRCGP.

Past papers   The Exam Regulations contain comprehensive examples of the type of questions asked in the written and MCQ papers. Books purporting to be 'sample questions' for both papers are published commercially, but most antedate the modularisation of the exam and should be treated with caution. The full text of the written paper is published on the RCGP website (www.rcgp.org.uk) shortly after each sitting of the exam, and a composite sample MCQ paper is made available at regular intervals for revision purposes. A commentary on each module of the exam is also published on the website after each sitting. This is compiled by the Convenor of the module and contains an appraisal of how the latest cohort of candidates have performed. It is a valuable source of guidance for future candidates.

Courses   A number of organisations offer preparatory courses on a commercial basis, including the RCGP at both national and faculty levels. Many potential candidates clearly find them helpful or at least reassuring. I confess to a personal scepticism, however. Usually, little material is provided that is not freely available, either from the College itself or already in the public domain. Some candidates might find the opportunity for group discussion of written paper topics, or of mock orals, useful. There is, however, a danger that participants confuse learning about the exam with preparing for it. I know of no evidence attesting to the 'value-added' merits of attending preparation courses, although (as your critical appraisal skills should confirm) absence of evidence is not the same as evidence of absence.

My personal advice is that the best and most cost-effective means of preparing specifically for the exam, aside from the foregoing, is to organise local study groups in which you cooperate with your peers in discussing clinical problems and practice issues, and answering questions from recent exams.

Pitfalls   The most common pitfall into which candidates preparing for the MRCGP fall is over-reliance on what they think to be good exam technique. The danger is to confuse technique with substance; to hope that a highly structured answer will be marked as if it was highly competent, that cliché and jargon will be mistaken for true comprehension. In the written paper, for example, some candidates' answers are formulaic to the point of being almost comic. Every patient, allegedly, has his or her Ideas, Concerns and Expectations explored. Every issue apparently has implications for the Patient, the Doctor, the Family, the Practice, the Team, Society, the Universe… No problem, it seems, is beyond the involvement of the Health Visitor, no ethical dilemma unworthy of reference to the doctor's defence organisation, no organisational matter too trivial to discuss at a full meeting of the Primary Health Care Team. A marking examiner, ears well attuned to the sound of an empty vessel, longs to say to the candidate, 'Tell me what you'd *really* do!'

A related condition is 'hyperquotosis' – larding every opinion or action with a plausible-sounding reference, 'As Thingummy showed, patients like you to know their name.' 'According to a recent paper by So-and-so, doctors are opposed to premature death.'

Candidates preparing for the exam often arrange 'mock orals', or ask someone to comment on the video-tape they propose to submit. Although these can undeniably be helpful strategies, they are not without risks. Unless conducted by actual examiners, mock orals often lack the pace, focus and depth of real ones, and can give false reassurance. The performance criteria required to pass the video component are also quite specific and detailed (see Chapter 4), and many candidates have come to grief because someone unfamiliar with them has given a well-intentioned but ill-informed opinion that the tape ought to pass. You should make sure that you, and anyone whose advice you seek, such as your trainer, are fully acquainted with the current documentation – exam regulations and video workbook – supplied by the College. Bear in mind also that the opinion of one individual adviser might not be shared by the group of examiners who will be assessing your performance in the actual exam. To prevent possible disappointment or bad feeling, the Panel of Examiners are advised not to involve themselves in personal coaching or advising of individual candidates.

Finally …

Achieving the MRCGP is a significant challenge. However, if you set it as a goal early in your training, it can provide a practical focus during your time as a registrar, and represents a valuable testament to your effort and commitment.

Summary

- The MRCGP is currently a voluntary qualification, although this might change in the future.

- The Regulations for the MRCGP exam are a comprehensive and reliable guide to how the exam is conducted. They are updated annually and are available only from the Examination Department at the RCGP.

- There are four modules to the MRCGP: a written paper, a multiple choice paper, an assessment of consulting skills and an oral exam. You must pass all four modules to pass the exam but you can take the modules separately, if you want, over a period of 3 years.

- There is no fixed syllabus for the MRCGP, the content evolves as general practice itself evolves.

- Passing the MRCGP multiple choice paper exempts you from any knowledge-based summative assessment tests; passing the MRCGP video component exempts you from summative assessment tests of consulting skills. You can submit a single video-tape, which will first be assessed for the MRCGP and, if it fails this, fast-tracked through the summative assessment process.

- The MRCGP exam can be used as a practical focus during your time as a registrar.

References

Gardiner P, Chana N, Jones R 2001 An insider's guide to the MRCGP oral exam. Radcliffe Medical Press, Abingdon, Oxfordshire

Longmore JM, Wilkinson I, Torok E 2001 Oxford handbook of clinical medicine, 5th edn. Oxford University Press, Oxford

Moore R 2000 The MRCGP examination: a guide for candidates and teachers, 4th edn. The Royal College of General Practitioners, London

Palmer KT 1998 Notes for the MRCGP, 3rd edn. Blackwell Science, Oxford

Skelton J, Field S, Wiskin C, Tate P 1998 Those things you say … consultation skills and the RCGP examination. Radcliffe Medical Press, Abingdon, Oxfordshire

Vocational Training Summative Assessment Board 1998 Protocol for the management of summative assessment: statement by the Joint Committee on Postgraduate Training for General Practice RCGP, London

Useful contacts

Radcliffe Medical Press
18 Marcham Road
Abingdon
Oxfordshire OX14 1AA

Royal College of General Practitioners
The Examination Department
14 Princes Gate
London SW7 1PU
Tel: 020 7584 3165
Website: www.rcgp.org.uk

4 Consulting skills: learning and assessment

Roger Neighbour

Rarely will you find a chapter dealing with consulting skills – their nature, learning and assessment – in any book similar to this published outside the UK. It is a peculiarly British notion that the consultation between a doctor and a patient has its own unique dynamic, and requires of the doctor a repertoire of skills beyond the purely clinical. Why so?

The answer is probably a combination of historical accident and political expediency. The work of the Hungarian émigré Michael Balint in the 1950s made it legitimate for GPs to reflect on the psychological processes at work in their consultations (Balint 1957). The insights generated by the Balint school were enormously valuable in their own right; they have transformed the lives of countless patients and enhanced the self-esteem of participating doctors, who were sensitised to the subtleties of the relationship between themselves and the people who consult them.

Subsequent generations of British GPs, even if they have not devoted themselves single-mindedly to the discipline of the Balint tradition, have nevertheless tried systematically to analyse the components of a 'successful' consultation – one that cleanly, effectively and efficiently satisfies the agenda of both doctor and patient.

Efficiency in the consultation is very much at a premium in the UK, where, compared with other countries with universal access to primary care, consultation times are extremely short. A form of natural selection has operated to bring about the survival of those professional skills that help a doctor achieve speed and effectiveness without compromising safety, courtesy or respect for the patient as a person. Making diagnoses by hypothesis-testing and pattern recognition, rather than the exhaustive but time-consuming 'medical model' practised in hospitals, is one example. Managing the consultation process by mastery of its component communication skills is another.

A third strand contributing to the prominence of consulting skills in the curriculum of the registrar year is the system of vocational training itself, pioneered in the UK. In the 1970s, British general practice embarked on a systematic analysis of the array of knowledge and competences that underpinned good performance, so as to make them understandable and therefore learnable (RCGP 1972). Recognising the central role of the doctor–patient relationship, teachers of general practice applied the principle of 'analyse in order to teach' to the interpersonal and communication processes at work in the consultation. Several conceptual models of the consultation were developed, forming the basis of learning programmes and eventually of methods of assessment; they are summarised in this chapter.

What must be constantly borne in mind, however, is that consulting skills are techniques and not ends in themselves. Consultation models are means to ends, one of the most important being to make a reality of the virtue (often professed but less often practised) of patient-centredness.

Consultation models

The usual way of developing models of the consultation has been to observe apparently skilled practitioners at work, to differentiate the component 'micro-skills' they appear to use and to marshal these into descriptive lists and categories that can be studied and practised by learners. Pioneering work in this field was published in the 1970s by Patrick Byrne and Barrie Long, who analysed audio-tapes of over 2500 consultations (Byrne & Long 1976). They described six phases to the consultation:

- Phase I: the doctor establishes a relationship with the patient
- Phase II: the doctor discovers the reason for the patient's attendance
- Phase III: the doctor conducts a verbal and/or physical examination
- Phase IV: the doctor, or patient, or both consider the condition
- Phase V: the doctor and patient detail further management
- Phase VI: the doctor (usually) terminates the consultation.

Crucially for the development of subsequent consultation analysis, Byrne and Long recognised that common causes of dysfunctional consultations were insufficient attention being paid to Phases II and/or IV.

Three categories of consultation models can be discerned, although there is overlap between them:

1 *Tasks* – 'things to do', e.g. take a history, arrange further investigations. Task models often consist of lists of items and can be learned by rote from books or articles. The 'medical model' – history, examination, investigations, diagnosis, treatment – is the best known.

2 *Behaviours* – 'activities to be performed', e.g. greeting the patient, asking open-ended questions, giving explanations. Models emphasising behaviours lend themselves to being practised in training seminars and workshops, and are mainly concerned to develop the doctor's repertoire of skills.

3 *Outcomes* – 'goals to be achieved', e.g. establishing rapport, reaching shared understanding, discovering the patient's 'hidden agenda'. Models emphasising outcome are less concerned with whatever techniques the doctor might employ, as long as they produce the desired effect. Familiarity with 'outcome' models is best gained through formative feedback on the doctor's real-life performance, e.g. from a trainer sitting in on the consultation, or reviewing video recordings of actual consultations.

> **L** How do you usually conduct a consultation? Think about some recent consultation and try to identify the different phases and models you use.

An example of a relatively pure 'task' model is that set out by Stott and Davis in their 1979 paper *The exceptional potential in each primary care consultation*. They list four tasks:

1 management of presenting problem(s)
2 modification of help-seeking behaviours
3 management of continuing problems
4 opportunistic health promotion.

John Heron's *Six-category intervention analysis* (Heron 1975) is an example of a pure 'behaviour' model. (Heron developed this as a method of training counsellors but the skills it inculcates translate well into a general practice context.) Within an overall setting of concern for the patient's best interests, the doctor's interventions fall into one of six categories, each of which can be rehearsed separately before being integrated into an overall consulting style:

1 *Prescriptive* – giving advice or instructions
2 *Informative* – giving new information, instructions or options

3 *Confronting* – challenging inaccuracies, misunderstandings or erroneous beliefs
4 *Cathartic* – encouraging the release of emotion through crying, laughter or anger
5 *Catalytic* – encouraging the patient to discover and reveal his or her thoughts, concerns and feelings
6 *Supportive* – showing concern, offering reassurance and encouragement.

The consultation model coming closest to a pure 'outcome' one is that on which the MRCGP examination's video method of assessing consultation skills is based. The MRCGP method sets out 15 'performance criteria', which, taken as a whole, summate to the patient-centred consulting style expected of successful candidates (see p. 53). The criteria, for example 'encouraging the patient's contribution' or 'sharing management options with the patient', specify what outcomes or goals should be achieved, but do not prescribe how this is to be done.

Most of the consultation models in current prominence are 'mixed', combining task, behaviour and outcome elements in varying proportions. The first such mixed model was set out by Pendleton et al in their 1984 book *The consultation: an approach to learning and teaching.* They detail seven 'tasks' for the consultation:

1 To define the reason for the patient's attendance (including what has, unfortunately, become a cliché parroted by exam candidates – the patient's Ideas, Concerns and Expectations)
2 To consider other problems, including risk factors
3 With the patient, to choose an appropriate action for each problem
4 To achieve a shared understanding of the problems with the patient
5 To involve the patient in the management and encourage him or her to accept appropriate responsibility
6 To use time and resources appropriately
7 To establish or maintain a relationship with the patient that helps achieve the other tasks.

Pendleton et al (1984) also suggest a robust system of skills training in which teacher and pupil contract to undertake a learning cycle, making extensive use of video review, role play and assessment checklists.

In his 1987 book *The inner consultation*, Neighbour explicitly differentiated the task, behaviour and outcome components. He identified five 'checkpoints' to be sequentially reached in the consultation:

1 *Connecting* – building a working rapport with the patient
2 *Summarizing* – being able to show that the doctor has correctly understood the patient's agenda
3 *Handover* – negotiating and communicating an acceptable strategy for managing the patient's concerns
4 *Safety-netting* – anticipating future developments and actions

5 *Housekeeping* – maintaining the doctor's own equanimity, equilibrium and emotional well-being.

Neighbour (1987) describes a wide range of 'micro-skills' that can be deployed in gaining each checkpoint, and which can be practised either in formal training sessions or within real-life consultations. He also encourages the doctor to cultivate a focused awareness of cues coming from the patient, which help to keep the consultation process on track and to ensure that the subtleties of the patient's agenda and reactions are picked up.

In 1998, two linked books by Silverman, Kurtz and Draper (Silverman et al 1998, Kurtz et al 1998) brought to the UK a communication skills training programme based on their experience of primary care in Canada and described as an agenda-led outcome-based analysis. In their 'Calgary–Cambridge observation guide' they listed five component tasks for the consultation:

1 initiating the session
2 gathering information
3 building the relationship
4 explanation and planning
5 closing the session.

These broad elements are further broken down into 70 constituent skills, which can be acquired separately through study and rehearsal before being integrated into a seamless whole.

The Calgary–Cambridge model is predominantly 'behavioural': Silverman et al (1998) describe each micro-skill in detail; Kurtz et al (1998) provide resource material for a programme of group- and video-based teaching.

The doctor's communication handbook (Tate 1994) (one of the et al in the Pendleton book and, from 2002, Convenor of the MRCGP Examination) deserves mention here. Tate is suitably eclectic in his account of the consultation process and to read his book comes close to attending a master class in communication with a genuine enthusiast.

Learning strategies

In fact, enthusiasm and its close relative curiosity are probably the main qualities that all the authors in this field are seeking to instil in GPs at the outset of their careers. If you are a relative newcomer to general practice, the choice of which consultation model to work with is relatively unimportant: you should be guided by your own preference for a particular approach or style, and by your own trainer's experience. Moreover, you should not rely on any digest or potted version of the consultation literature – not even the present chapter. Acquiring a command of the consultation process is so fundamental an element of modern general practice that I believe you should pay it the respect of going to the original source material in all its richness. What matters supremely is that, right from the start of your training, you should discover that there is such a thing as being good at consulting, which is separate from and additional to the various clinical and organisational skills you need to acquire. You are unlikely to find practice as satisfying as it could be unless you can take pride and pleasure in improving your own consulting skills. This means being unafraid to submit your work to scrutiny – your own initially, your trainer's, your peers', and ultimately that of summative assessment and the MRCGP examination. You can achieve a certain amount through private reflection and through case discussion. But the dangers of self-deception and collusion always exist unless you are willing to take as the raw material for your education the hard evidence of what actually transpires in your everyday consultations, and that inescapably means using video. The most important single step you can take towards becoming proficient in the art of consulting is to overcome camera-shyness and to make regular video recordings of your surgeries throughout your training year. Your trainer will no doubt offer tutorials on various aspects of the consultation process and you will have the opportunity of attending workshops and seminars on the subject. But video recording has transformed the process of improving communication skills and is something to be welcomed as an everyday tool of the trade.

Making video recordings of your consultations

The commonly expressed reservation – that 'I won't perform naturally in front of the camera' – quickly evaporates with familiarity. The technical requirements for successful video recording of consultations are not complicated, but they are important.

Equipment

It is sensible to use equipment that records in a format that can later be used to submit your work for summative assessment and the MRCGP. At present, you have to submit in standard VHS format, recorded at normal speed (not long play). If you use a VHS-C or other small format camcorder, make sure you have the facilities to transcribe onto a standard VHS cassette. Tapes submitted for summative assessment might need the time and date to be superimposed on the recording.

The built-in microphones on many camcorders give poor quality sound reproduction, tending to amplify background noise disproportionately, to the disadvantage of the spoken (often softly spoken) words we are interested in. A separate desk-top wide-angle microphone discreetly positioned between doctor and patient gives much better results.

Camera position

Most modern camcorders give acceptable results in ordinary ambient lighting. Position the camera so that neither doctor nor patient is backlit against a window or bright light.

Intimate or sensitive examinations must be conducted 'off camera', either by positioning the camera suitably or by using a lens cap.

Most can be learned if the main 'communicative parts' of both doctor and patient, i.e. face, arms and upper body, are clearly visible. A camera positioned slightly above head height is least conspicuous, but you should ensure that facial expressions can be seen. A tripod can be used, but a wall-mounted bracket is less obtrusive.

Patient consent

The GMC has produced clear guidelines on using video recordings for educational and assessment purposes. Essentially, informed consent must be obtained in writing from the patient before and after recording. The consent form must state the purpose of the proposed recording, who will be allowed to view it and the arrangements for the tape's security. It must also be made clear that refusing consent will not disadvantage the patient. Suitable consent forms, which can be photocopied, are obtainable from Regional Deaneries and are included in the MRCGP video workbook.

Formative and summative assessment

An assessment intended to give non-judgemental feedback on the learner's performance and to provide a 'steer' on future learning is said to be 'formative'. An assessment made with the intention of passing judgement, particularly if a 'pass/fail' decision is involved, is called 'summative'. Video (and indeed most other assessment modalities) can be used either formatively or summatively: you can make video recordings either to improve and fine-tune your skills by being alerted to your strengths and weaknesses, or as a portfolio of evidence of your performance submitted for a significant career milestone.

Some people feel there is an irreconcilable tension between the two purposes. 'How can you perform naturally,' they ask, 'if you are afraid to show your weakness for fear of failure?' I think this is an unnecessary concern, for two reasons. First, the aspects of your consulting ability that you will study formatively are no different from those used summatively by assessors and examiners. Second, you always have the option of not submitting for assessment any recordings you are not satisfied with.

Using video formatively

You have made a tape of one of your surgeries: how can you best learn from it?

> **L** Have you made any video recordings of your consultations? The earlier you start to do this, the more you will learn and the better your performance during consultations (and in the video part of summative assessment or the MRCGP exam).

It may be that you have decided in advance to review one particular aspect of your communication skills, such as your use of open-ended questions or jargon, or body language and other non-verbal communication. Or you and your trainer might have a predetermined educational goal linked to one or other of the formal consultation models described earlier. But I believe you can get most from watching yourself on video-tape if you do so dispassionately and in an unstructured way, without too many preconceptions, as if the doctor on the screen was a stranger whom you were observing quite neutrally. Some of the questions you might find yourself asking are:

- Does the consultation get off to a good start? If not, why not?
- What is it about this doctor's style that takes my attention?
- Does the doctor have any irritating or distracting mannerisms?
- Does the doctor seem genuinely interested in the patient? If not, how can I tell?
- Is there a real rapport between the two?
- Does the consultation seem to run to a set formula? If so, is it helpful?
- Is the doctor paying attention to what is going on?
- What seems to matter most to this patient?
- Is the doctor picking up on cues to the patient's hidden agenda? If not, how can I tell?
- Whose agenda seems to be the more important?
- What can I tell from the body language and eye contact of doctor and patient?
- Are doctor and patient using language that both can understand?
- Do the doctor's contributions seem to help or hinder those of the patient?
- Does the doctor seem to understand the patient's own perception of the problem?
- Does the doctor's use of the notes or the computer ever get in the way of the consultation process?
- What do I think of the doctor's clinical judgement and decision-making? Have the right possibilities been considered?
- Does the patient seem to understand and be satisfied with what is being said? If not, how can I tell?
- Who seems to be controlling the consultation? Doctor or patient, or is it a shared responsibility?
- Does the consultation come to an appropriate end? If not, why not, and how can I tell?

Questions like these, although they do not necessarily form part of one consultation model rather than another, nevertheless raise your aware-ness of what is going on in such a way that you might be able to iden-tify areas of your performance that could do with improving. Getting into the habit of asking them will cultivate an attitude of mind that is genuinely curious about what is going on in the consultation and about the dynamics operating between doctor and patient, which is what being patient-centred means. Looking at yourself on video provides a 'credibility and genuineness check'. If you do this regularly, you need have little to fear from submitting samples of your work for any form of summative assessment.

Using video summatively

Submitting a video-tape of your consultations is one of several methods of demonstrating your 'ability to consult effectively with general practice patients' as required for the purposes of summative assessment. (Non-video methods, such as those using simulated patients, are not considered here.) Video is also, to all intents and purposes, the method you will take as the consulting skills component of the MRCGP examination. (Very few registrar candidates will be eligible to take the College's alternative of simulated surgery, which is at present reserved for people having insuperable difficulty in submitting a video-tape.)

Those involved in administering summative assessment and the MRCGP have been well aware of the workload involved for registrars who, having to prepare a video for summative assessment, also had to submit a tape made to different specifications if they elected to sit the Membership exam. Since 2001, therefore, provision has been made to allow candidates for both assessments to submit a single tape. The tape is marked first by MRCGP video examiners, and if successful for Membership will be deemed also to have passed for summative assessment purposes. If unsuccessful for Membership, the tape will (if the candidate has so requested) be fast-tracked through the summative assessment marking process. Because the requirements for summative assessment are less stringent than those for MRCGP, about 90% of 'single-track' tapes that fail the RCGP method will go on to pass summative assessment.

The regulations governing the submission of tapes for summative assessment, the MRCGP and the single-track option are detailed, precise, might vary from year to year, and will be strictly adhered to. This chapter will therefore only indicate broad principles. *You **must** make sure that you obtain up-to-date information from your Regional Deanery and/or the RCGP Examination Department.* Failure to do so may jeopardise your success.

Summative assessment

For the purposes of summative assessment registrars must demonstrate that, to a level of 'minimum competence', they can:

- identify the reasons for the patient's attendance
- take appropriate steps to investigate the problems presented
- organise a suitable management plan
- reach an agreement with the patient on diagnosis and treatment
- demonstrate an understanding (by documenting it in a logbook) of what was going on in the consultation.

The registrar must show positive evidence of these skills and must therefore submit consultations with a sufficient degree of challenge to allow them to be demonstrated. Tapes are assessed under the headings of Listening, Action and Understanding. In addition, dangerous or cumulative errors of clinical judgement seen on the tape might lead to its being referred for further scrutiny or possible failure.

The MRCGP video assessment

The MRCGP methodology incorporates the common features of the best-known consultation models, refined by reference to a broadly based panel of examiners, trainers, educationists and lay representatives. The College unashamedly expects its Members to be able to consult in a patient-centred style, all the research evidence being that this correlates best with good clinical outcomes and patient satisfaction. These values are expressed in 15 performance criteria' (PCs) against which tapes submitted for the MRCGP exam are appraised. (For accurate and up-to-date information on the procedure for submitting tapes, as well as advice on how to prepare and details of how tapes are marked, you *must* refer to the Regulations and Video Workbook provided by the RCGP Examination Department (see the Useful contacts section at the end of this chapter). Essentially, you submit a tape of seven consultations, which you have selected. The examiners will look for evidence of Membership-level competence in each PC on up to four occasions in the seven consultations.)

The 15 PCs are themselves derived from the following composite model of the consultation, set out and explained in the Video Workbook.

- *Discover the reasons for a patient's attendance:*
  - elicit the patient's account of the symptom(s) that made him/her turn to the doctor
  - obtain relevant items of social and occupational circumstances
  - explore the patient's health understanding
  - enquire about continuing problems

- *Define the clinical problem(s):*
  - obtain additional information about symptoms and details of medical history
  - access the condition of the patient by appropriate physical or mental examination
  - make a working diagnosis

- *Explain the problem(s) to the patient:*
  - share the findings with the patient
  - tailor the explanation to the patient
  - ensure that the explanation is understood and accepted by the patient

- *Address the patient's problem(s):*
  - access the severity of the presenting problem(s)
  - choose an appropriate form of management
  - involve the patient in the management plan to an appropriate extent

■ *Make effective use of the consultation:*
  – make efficient use of resources
  – establish a relationship with the patient
  – give opportunistic health promotion advice.

The performance criteria

Competence in all of the 12 PCs marked (*P*) in the following list must be demonstrated to pass. The three marked (*M*) are 'merit' PCs; if you pass these as well as the others you will be awarded a 'pass with merit' in the video module.

1 (*P*) The doctor encourages the patient's contribution at appropriate points in the consultation
2 (*P*) The doctor responds to cues
3 (*P*) The doctor elicits appropriate details to place the complaint(s) in a social and psychological context
4 (*M*) The doctor takes the patient's health understanding into account
5 (*P*) The doctor obtains sufficient information for no serious condition to be missed
6 (*P*) The doctor chooses an examination that is likely to confirm or disprove hypotheses that could reasonably have been formed *or* to address the patient's concern
7 (*P*) The doctor appears to make a clinically appropriate working diagnosis
8 (*P*) The doctor explains the diagnosis, management and effects of treatment
9 (*P*) The doctor explains in language appropriate to the patient
10 (*M*) The doctor's explanation takes account of some or all of the patient's health beliefs
11 (*M*) The doctor seeks to confirm the patient's understanding
12 (*P*) The doctor's management plan is appropriate for the working diagnosis, reflecting a good understanding of modern accepted medical practice
13 (*P*) The doctor shares the management options with the patient
14 (*P*) The doctor's prescribing behaviour is appropriate
15 (*P*) The patient and doctor appear to have established a rapport.

Discussion of the MRCGP video assessment

That the MRCGP model of the consultation and the PCs derived from it look familiar to you by now should come as no surprise. After all, they represent the commonly agreed tasks, behaviours and outcomes that make for efficient patient-centred consulting. Nevertheless, the video assessment has the highest failure rate of all the examination's modules (about 25%). There are some important points of emphasis that you need to understand if you are to get the most out of the effort you will be putting into your formative and summative use of video.

The philosophy of the MRCGP video is that outcome matters more than process. As the Video Workbook makes clear, the PCs are not to be taken in isolation but as interlocking components of a holistic view of what skilled consulting consists of, namely the doctor bringing all his or her professional skills to the service of the patient. An analogy with the driving test (quoted in the MRCGP Examiners' training manual!) may make this clearer.

To pass the test, you have to 'turn the car to face the opposite direction, using forward and reverse gears, safely, without endangering other road users, nor striking the kerb or other obstacles'. The number of forward/reverse iterations is not specified, neither is there a time limit, but the examiner would expect the manoeuvre to be carried out with a certain smoothness. Clearly many skills are involved (clutch control, spatial awareness, steering etc.) But ultimately there is one over-riding outcome to be achieved – getting the car to point the other way.

Research within the MRCGP Panel of Examiners has shown that the ability to consult regularly in a patient-centred way is relatively slow to develop. Few registrars are able to demonstrate it consistently by the end of their training year (although most can after they have been in practice a year or two more) (Tate, personal communication, 2001). For this reason, the MRCGP allows and expects candidates to 'cherry-pick' the consultations they choose for submission and to put together a video portfolio of their best material to show the examiners. The principle is the same as an apprentice cabinetmaker discarding early, botched efforts and preparing a 'masterpiece' of best work to submit for a graduation assessment.

MRCGP candidates have more difficulty with some performance criteria than others (Campion et al 2002). Analysis of data to 2000 showed that PC11 (confirming the patient's understanding) was shown twice or more in the tapes of only 23% of candidates, and PC13 (sharing management options) was found twice or more in only 36%. Many candidates also found picking-up on a patient's hidden agenda (PC2, 'responding to cues') hard to demonstrate.

There could be many reasons for these rather discouraging findings. Assessment methods inevitably operate at some remove from real life, although using video comes closer than most alternatives. The fear of making a blunder on tape makes some candidates submit only 'low challenge' consultations, which do not provide an opportunity to display higher-order consulting skills. Others leave it until late in their training before starting to collect potential video material, and find themselves spending large amounts of time trying to collect suitable consultations. There is also a correlation between registrars' success in the consulting skills assessment and their trainers' personal familiarity with the consultation literature in general and the MRCGP methodology in particular. The MRCGP video pass rate is highest in Regions where

Deans, Course Organisers and trainers have taken this on board (Tate, personal communication, 2001).

Nevertheless, it is clear that skill in consulting is something that has to be worked at. The best advice is 'start early.' Make the acquaintance of some of the consultation literature early in your vocational training. Take any opportunity to go on consulting skills courses and seminars. Get quickly into the habit of making frequent video recordings of your consultations, so that you overcome the inevitable diffidence and can begin to make good formative use of the technology. Regularly appraise your own performance with the various checklists, models and assessment tools. That way you will come to appreciate that being good at consulting brings its own rewards, and that acquiring the necessary skills can deepen your understanding of the personal nature of general practice.

Summary

- The work of Michael Balint, in the 1950s, began the search for what makes a 'successful' consultation between patient and doctor.

- Byrne and Long (1976) described six phases to a consultation.

- From this, three models of consultation were identified: task-based, behaviour-based and outcome-based. Most consultations combine elements of these three models.

- However, enthusiasm and curiosity are probably the main qualities necessary for a 'successful' consultation.

- Video recordings can help registrars to analyse their own consultation style and improve on areas of weakness.

- Video tapes submitted for the MRCGP exam are measured against 15 performance criteria.

References

Balint M 1957 The doctor, his patient and the illness. Tavistock Publications, London

Byrne PS, Long BEL 1976 Doctors talking to patients. HMSO, London

Campion P, Tate P, Foulkes J, Neighbour R 2002 Patient-centredness is rare among candidates in the MRCGP video examination: an analysis of 2096 doctors and 14,852 consultations (in preparation)

Heron J 1975 Six-category intervention analysis. Human Potential Resource Group, Guildford, Surrey

Kurtz S, Silverman J Draper J 1998 Teaching and learning communication skills in medicine. Radcliffe Medical Press, Abingdon, Oxfordshire

Neighbour R 1987 The inner consultation. Petroc Press, Newbury, Berkshire

Pendleton D, Schofield T, Tate P, Havelock P 1984 The consultation: an approach to learning and teaching. Oxford University Press, Oxford

RCGP 1972 The future general practitioner: learning and teaching. Report of the Working Party of the Royal College of General Practitioners. Royal College of General Practitioners, London

Silverman J, Kurtz S, Draper J 1998 Skills for communicating with patients. Radcliffe Medical Press, Abingdon, Oxfordshire

Stott NCH, Davis RH 1979 The exceptional potential in each primary care consultation. Journal of the Royal College of General Practitioners 29:201–205

Tate P 1994 The doctor's communication handbook. Radcliffe Medical Press, Abingdon, Oxfordshire

Useful addresses

Royal College of General Practitioners
The Examination Department
14 Princes Gate
London SW7 1PU
Tel: 020 7584 3165
Website: www.rcgp.org.uk

5 Health, illness and disease: a general practice perspective

Surinder Singh

As a medical student, you probably learnt something along the lines of 'illness is what a patient has when they go to the doctor and disease is what they have when they leave' (Helman 1998). This chapter will examine the concepts of illness and disease in the context of general practice. Ideas from the relatively recent disciplines of medical anthropology and the medical humanities will be introduced to suggest new perspectives in our understanding of these very basic ideas in health care.

Definitions of illness and disease

We know that a patient's experience of illness is different from a doctor's understanding of disease. But why do we need these different ways of describing the same thing? In biomedicine, defined as the collective knowledge that assumes a scientific and technical basis for many conditions, disease and illness are intimately connected. Thus, for example, a 55-year-old woman who falls and fractures a wrist and experiences pain. The patient's illness in this case will be fairly consistent with her disease – that being the fracture of the wrist and perhaps a degree of underlying osteoporosis. As the healing then takes place the pain diminishes, movements start to improve and, some time, later the wrist returns more or less to normal. But it is not that simple.

Let us think about the cultural group this woman comes from. Would it make a difference, for example, if she was born and bred in London or if she originated from Mauritius? What are the underlying beliefs of the woman regarding the fall that caused the fracture? How likely is it that the Londoner believes that a 'spell has been cast', causing her to fall by way of punishment for some past deed?

What about illness without disease?

In general practice you will soon get to know many patients who have an illness but no disease (Helman 1981). This is where the doctor needs to use all his or her skill to acknowledge the experience of the patient and yet communicate that there is no serious medical problem. It is part of our job to assess people presenting with non-specific, often self-limiting conditions that might then require very little input apart from a sensible explanation and a degree of reassurance. This role of excluding serious pathology and providing reassurance is a valuable one and should not be taken lightly. We all develop our ways of explaining self-limiting conditions which are bad when around (e.g. a nasty dose of flu) but which disappear without any significant medical interventions (Helman 1978).

And disease without illness?

Disease without illness is also a common scenario and has been a fairly modern phenomenon since the advent of medical diagnostic techniques (Helman 1998). Cervical cancer screening or blood pressure testing fall into this category. Although they are done for positive reasons, they clearly (in many cases) give people disease before they experience illness. This can have important consequences. For example, in the case of moderate hypertension, some patients will not take medication because they feel perfectly well, if not better, without it.

Case illustrations

> Think of these common presentations in general practice – are these examples of illness or disease?
>
> - A 35-year-old pregnant woman returns to see the GP fairly early in the first trimester wanting advice. She is very worried about a 'little pain' she had earlier in the day which has now settled.
> - A 50-year-old man, previously an engineer, consults about an intermittent but longstanding headache for the past 8 years following a work-related accident. He takes regular simple analgesic but 'wants something stronger'.
> - A 60-year-old woman presents with 'excessive wind' with no other symptoms whatsoever – in fact she tells you 'she is quite fit'.

Models

Models are simply a way of seeing the world – perhaps a reminder of things that are simple, familiar and instantly recognisable. They can also be seen as a representation of something more complex and it is in this context that models can be used to help us understand illness and its implications, and also to analyse doctor–patient interactions. Some of these explanatory models are discussed in the following pages. It is important to be aware of their existence but not to be weighed down by them (Neighbour 1987).

The biomedical model of illness and disease

Diagnosis lies at the heart of the biomedical model of illness and disease but what are the other features of this model (Good 1994, Helman 1998)?

- The human body is composed of different organs, all of which are interconnected in some special way. Because much is now known about the anatomy, biochemistry and physiology of such a complex system, it is as if the whole is more than the sum of its constituent parts.
- Diseases are processes that cause deviation in the working of the overall structure, such that an organ or organs begin to work suboptimally.
- Pathology is the study of this aberration in whatever form it takes, be it anatomical, biochemical or physiological.
- A patient's problem is due to the above aberration, which is manifest in signs and symptoms, and it is the doctor's role to try and highlight where this is through the process of diagnosis.
- Once a diagnosis has been made a management plan can be put in place designed to reverse the changes brought about by the aberration identified earlier.

Other models of illness

There are many other models of illness (McWhinney 1997, Neighbour 1987, Pendleton et al 1984). For example:

- the sociological model
- the psychoanalytical model
- the health-belief model
- the sociopolitical model
- the behavioural model.

All of these models add together to give us the real picture of why a particular patient presents to a doctor. Although medical training equips us well to apply the biomedical model, each of the other perspectives has something to contribute to our understanding and each can highlight deficiencies in the traditional Western medical model.

Another way of looking at things is provided by the anthropological approach. A particular advantage of medical anthropology is that it attempts to incorporate many of the other models into one overarching representation (Good 1994, Helman 1998, Horder 2001).

The consultation

The consultation is a place where all of these models of health and illness can potentially be put into action (see Chapter 4). Indeed, for each model of illness there is a corresponding model of the consultation (Neighbour 1987, Pendleton et al 1984) and each of these provides us with insights into why patients present and the various processes that make up the consultation. The role of the doctor, his or her level of interpersonal skills and how they are used, how the doctor responds to the patient and the doctor's own feelings all influence the consultation (Pendleton et al 1984).

You might think that the doctor–patient meeting is functional, because patients know when to consult doctors and doctors know what patients want from these consultations. Unfortunately, this is often not the case. About 1 million GP consultations occur every day within the UK NHS, and research has shown that patients and doctors do not always see eye-to-eye about the nature of these consultations.

An anthropological model of the consultation

Cecil Helman was the first GP to look at how, in many ways, the doctor in the West was similar to a traditional healer in the East or to a Shaman in the South (Helman 1998). All are supposed to have 'healing' properties, bestowed upon them by their indigenous cultures, and all have various trappings of this 'power' on show. In the West, this property is only 'bestowed' after a fairly arduous training. Think of the average doctor's surgery and the symbols of the doctor that will be displayed for all to see – bleep, stethoscope, otoscope, medical posters, maybe degrees on display – and it will be clear who the professional is and what they do.

Helman described six questions that encompassed the patient's attempts to work out why they had fallen 'ill' (Box 5.1). Illness here can refer to anything from unwanted symptoms (or signs) through to bad luck and acts of 'nature'.

These questions form a type of explanatory model of the ideas, perceptions and beliefs regarding a particular illness episode. Often these beliefs are idiosyncratic, everchanging and may be completely different to the doctor's understanding.

Going to the doctor

What is it that makes patients come to doctors? McWhinney and many others have shown that, in fact, of all the people in any community, only

Box 5.1
The anthropological approach

1 What has happened?
2 Why has it happened?
3 Why to me?
4 Why now?
5 What would happen if nothing were done about it?
6 What should I do about it or whom should I consult for further help?

a small percentage will visit the doctor when they feel unwell (McWhinney 1997). There are many reasons why individuals don't come: domestic commitments, getting away from work and difficulties in making appointments are just three common reasons. Nevertheless, studies in the developed world have shown that, in the average locality, about three-quarters of all adults will have 'symptoms', that is, will have perceived something to be wrong, during the previous 2 weeks. Even here there is some difficulty with nomenclature – it is easy for doctors to see patients' problems as 'symptoms', but remember that for the patient it is just 'I am feeling unwell or not my usual self'. Therefore, of 1000 people in the community, 750 will have such symptoms at any one time. About one-third of these (approximately 250) will report to a clinician, which already means that the majority will avoid the doctor. Of the 250 who consult, five will be referred to another clinician and about 10 will be referred to hospital. These figures are one of the reasons behind the 'iceberg of illness' that is prevalent in the community. In other words, doctors see only a small percentage of people who are ill or sick (McWhinney 1997).

Below is a selection of broad reasons why patients consult (Helman 1998):

- *Perceived changes in body appearance* – weight-loss or gain
- *Unusual body emissions* – urinary frequency, or abnormal menstruation
- *Changes in the senses* – deafness, problems with sight, numbness, pain
- *Emotional states* – anxiety, depression, nightmares, other concerns
- *Behavioural changes* – in relation to family, work, pleasure.

Case illustration

> A 40-year-old woman with previously diagnosed diabetes mellitus returned to the doctor with weight loss, which she recognised as being a symptom that should be checked out. Closer questioning revealed her to be non-compliant (or non-concordant) with advice and medication.
>
> - Is this an illness or disease?
> - Does it matter?
> - Does the illness–disease approach affect your management decisions?

Medical anthropology as another way of seeing the world

Medical anthropology is a relatively new discipline that has grown out of social anthropology. It is one of the fastest growing subdisciplines in North American universities and aims to explore the cultural aspects of health in a global world. Although many definitions exist, its prime objective is to explore, in a humanistic way, various influences on the health of a person, family, village or community unit, however that is defined. At least one definition cites the biocultural understanding of humans and their works in relation to health and medicine (Van der Geest & Rienks 1998). Wider definitions exist; for example, some think that medical anthropology is that branch of applied anthropology that deals with various aspects of health and disease (Van der Geest & Rienks 1998). It encompasses many specialties, from biomedicine through to sociology, psychology, women's studies and geography, as well as economics, politics and history, and is truly holistic – in a way that medicine is most definitely not. In many ways it attempts to combine all the models cited above and to produce one that is truly reflective of what is really happening to people, families and communities.

How is this related to medicine and general practice? This is where you need to look at medicine in its broadest sense – all the way from its basic availability, through to its functions and how it treats patients and people, including its practitioners. Ultimately, it is patients who ought to be judging medicine's skills, processes and outcomes; however, along the way politics and economics have to be factored in because success often depends on the amount of resources health care has been allocated – again a political decision in many parts of the world. All of this is encompassed by medical anthropology, although how this can be applied needs the skills of many disciplines, including researchers, patient advocates, practitioners, local community representatives and more.

Thus, going to the GP for any particular patient is as much about the process (for example, who did they talk to before coming?) as it is about the 'consultation'. What happened during this meeting – was the doctor kind, listening and empathic, or did he or she interrupt, appear not to listen and write out a prescription as the patient sat down? And what about the advice given to the patient from the others in the waiting room? And finally, the patient's actions after seeing the doctor are as much part of this process as anything else. In other words, the patient's intention of going to casualty in another day or two if the problem does not settle is as important as the meeting with the doctor. This last scenario might include the visit the patient is intending to make to see the herbal therapist or the *Tai Chi* specialist once the appointment is over. All of this – the various elements that make up the person who is 'ill' and the acts of seeking advice – is studied by medical anthropologists.

Is there too much medicine?

A special edition of the *British Medical Journal* in 2002 explored in detail the merits or otherwise of categorising various conditions as diseases or non-diseases (Moynihan & Smith 2002). The edition questioned whether normal events and processes, such as pregnancy, birth, pain, old age and dying, have been so medicalised as to do more harm than good in society? In this same issue of the *BMJ*, several commentators argued about the growing list of non-diseases (for example 'bags under eyes', 'boredom' or 'baldness') and diseases; even for the latter the boundaries are often unclear. The fact is that many of the terms we take for granted in discussions of health, illness and disease are poorly defined, inconsistent, blurred or even slippery (Smith 2002). Political and financial motives, for example pharmaceutical companies marketing pills for 'lifestyle diseases', have their part to play in this situation. The challenge to general practice is to keep our patients' interests foremost in our minds in the light of all the competing issues and interests that impact on matters of health and illness.

A role for the medical humanities?

In recent years there has been a welter of books, newspaper articles and television programmes on the experiences of being ill. Why is this? Is it not paradoxical that as technology in medicine progresses, clinicians seem to be viewed with more suspicion and concern. Some would even say that a crisis is at hand (Heath 1995, Helman 1998, McWhinney 1997).

Part of this problem perhaps stems from a more general critical attitude in our society towards to all those in authority, including the professions. But our own training must surely bear some of the blame. Until relatively recently there was little emphasis on patients' experiences in undergraduate medical education. Think back to your own student days and try to remember how much (or little) time was spent learning about patients' lives, their family or their work compared to their symptoms, signs and pathophysiology. It is probably fair to say that the clinicians of say 50 years ago were in fact more experience-minded, perhaps because they could offer little to patients apart from themselves and a handful of stock medicines (Asher 1986). This is in sharp contrast to today; 10-min appointments, a burgeoning pharmacopoeia, endless tests to choose between and interpret, administration and perhaps that exam to prepare for all ensure that today's doctors are more harassed and almost certainly less patient-centred than they used to be. The result is that, despite our increased knowledge and technical ability, patients' overall experiences of health care are probably worse now than ever before.

Consider ...

What do you think of the current fashion for biographies (sometimes called 'pathographies') of individuals who have suffered serious, often eventually fatal illnesses (examples include the books by John Diamond, Ruth Picardie, Martin Harris and Robert McCrum). Is this a passing fad? What do these books tell us, as doctors, about the experience of illness and health care?

Humanistic medicine – rediscovered?

Whether coincidence or not, there has in recent years been a growing interest in the relationship between the humanities and medicine, both in terms of its academic contribution and its relationship to patient care. Several universities have established major interest groups, there is a new journal – the *Journal of Medical Humanities* – and several conferences have highlighted the growing role of the subspecialty. Why should this be so?

One argument is that this move is as a direct response to some of the factors that were highlighted above (Greenhalgh & Hurwitz 1998, Kirklin & Richardson 2001). There is a fear that medicine is becoming too technical, doctors are becoming more specialised (i.e. knowing more and more about less and less) and the patient's story – the basis of clinical medicine – is lost somewhere in the seemingly complex process that constitutes modern health care. The series called 'Personal views' in the *BMJ* often highlights the experiences of health professionals as patients themselves. These short articles point to a malaise in the system that is not easily rectified (Anon 1999, Easterbrooke 1999, McCall 1999).

One of the reasons people go to the doctor is to articulate concerns, share experiences and engage with an 'interested other' who might be able to help in some way. We hear a lot more today about patients' 'narrative' – the 'story' behind their presentation. This might be the most important aspect of a doctor–patient consultation and certainly underlies Balint's way of looking at some of the intractable problems patients bring to doctors (Balint 1964).

Much of this has been encapsulated by the notion of narrative-based medicine, in which the importance of the patient's story takes centre-stage in the doctor–patient relationship (Heath 1995). Although many would think that this approach is the antithesis of evidence-based medicine, the pragmatist would see both of these notions as complementary. If evidence-based medicine is based purely on 'medical evidence' then medicine becomes fairly autocratic and paternal, whereas putting into practice evidence or guidelines can – and should – always take the patient's view into account. This is what is probably meant by the 'art' of medicine.

Summary

This chapter has looked at several topics under the terms 'health' and 'illness'. Understanding the meaning of these concepts and how they relate to the whole range of people we see, with their various problems, is what makes general practice perhaps the most challenging of specialties. The recent interest in models other than the traditional biomedical model, in medical anthropology, narrative-based medicine and medical humanities perhaps results from a crisis of confidence in medicine. Technological advances and political pressures have shifted the focus away from the patient as a person but patients want and need humanistic, compassionate and clinically competent doctors who are knowledgeable, can interpret information in all sorts of ways and have the ability to transmit this back in an understandable way to the patient. It is a tall order, but then being a good doctor always has been.

■ Looking afresh at the concepts of illness and disease makes us realise that patients and doctors do not always talk the same language. Acknowledging this is the first step in attempting to be more patient-centred – an increasingly important approach if we are to enhance the patient's involvement in decision-making.

- It is easy to forget the story of the patient's visit to the doctor, and perhaps this is one of the reasons why the patient narrative has become more fashionable and prominent recently.

- Both the medical humanities and, in particular, medical anthropology are specialties that enable us to see the world in a much wider, more relevant context. We hope this benefits you but especially your patients.

L Are you tempted, on reading this synopsis of medical philosophy, sociology and anthropology, to ask 'Does it all matter? Is it relevant to what I have to do day-by-day in the surgery?' The answer to this question is an emphatic 'Yes!'

An inquisitive doctor is a thoughtful doctor, and a thoughtful doctor is a good doctor. If for no other reason, having a sense of cultural perspective on the work you do is a good antidote to frustration and burn-out. What's more, being able to articulate some of these ideas will stimulate you to think more laterally when answering questions in the written paper, and gives you the chance to lift your performance in the oral exams to meritorious levels.

References

Anon 1999 'In memory of Annie' – personal view. British Medical Journal 318:745

Asher R 1986 Talking sense, 1st edn. Churchill Livingstone, London

Balint M 1964 The doctor, his patient and the illness, 2nd edn. Pitman Press, London

Easterbrooke J 1999 'The emperor has no clothes on' – personal view. British Medical Journal 318:473

Good B 1994 Medicine rationality and experience: an anthropological perspective. Cambridge University Press, Cambridge

Greenhalgh T, Hurwitz B 1998 Narrative-based medicine, 1st edn. BMJ Books, London

Heath I 1995 The mystery of general practice, 1st edn. The Nuffield Provincial Hospitals Trust, London

Helman C 1978 'Feed and cold, starve a fever': folk models of infection in an English suburban community, and their relation to medical treatment. Culture, Medicine and Psychiatry 2:107–137

Helman C 1981 Disease versus illness in general practice. Journal of the Royal College of General Practitioners 31:548–552

Helman C 1998 Culture, health and illness, 4th edn. Butterworth-Heinemann, Oxford

Horder J 2001 The first Balint group. British Journal of General Practice 51(473):1038–1039

Kirklin D, Richardson R 2001 Medical humanities: a practical introduction. Royal College of Physicians Publishing, London

McCall K 1999 'An insider's guide to depression' – personal view. British Medical Journal 318:745

McWhinney I 1997, A textbook of family medicine, 2nd edn. Oxford University Press, New York

Moynihan R, Smith R 2002 Editorial: too much medicine? British Medical Journal 324:859–860

Neighbour R 1987 The inner consultation, 1st edn. Kluwer Academic Publications, Dordrecht

Pendleton D, Schofield T, Tate P et al 1984 The consultation: an approach to learning and teaching (Oxford GP series No. 6), 1st edn. Oxford Publications, Oxford

Smith R 2002 In search of 'non-disease'. British Medical Journal 324:883–885

Van der Geest S, Rienks A (eds) 1998 The art of medical anthropology: readings, 1st edn. Het Spinhuis Publishers, Amsterdam

Further reading

Asher R 1986 Talking sense, 1st edn. Churchill Livingstone, London

Barsky AJ 1988 The paradox of health (special article). New England Journal of Medicine 318:414–418

Coulter A 2002 After Bristol: putting patients at the centre. British Medical Journal 324:648–651

Good B 1994 Medicine rationality and experience: an anthropological perspective. Cambridge University Press, Cambridge

Hahn R 1995 Sickness and healing, 1st edn. Yale University Press, New Haven, CT

Ibrahim S 2002 Editorial: the medicalisation of old age. British Medical Journal 324:861–863

Kleinman A 1995 Writing at the margin: discourse between anthropology and medicine. University of California Press, Berkeley, CA

Lloyd M, Bor R 1996 Communication skills for medicine, 1st edn. Churchill Livingstone, Edinburgh

Misselbrook D 2002 Thinking about patients. Petroc Press, London

Parsons T 1951 The social system. Free Press, New York

Schon D 1995 The reflective practitioner. Arena Press, Aldershot

Silverman J, Kurtz S, Draper J 1998 Skills for communicating with patients. Radcliffe Medical Press, Abingdon, Oxfordshire

Stevenson A (ed) 1998 A textbook of general practice. Arnold, London

Toon P 1999 Towards a philosophy of general practice: a study of the virtuous practitioner. RCGP Occasional paper no. 78. RCGP, London

Tuckett D, Boulton M, Olson C 1985 Meetings between experts. Tavistock Press, London

Useful contacts

The American Anthropological Association
www.aaanet.org/ar/
Big, useful and definitive – go and visit it.

The Society of Medical Anthropology
www.cudenver.edu//sma//index.html
The Society of Medical Anthropology is a subsection of the larger and extremely diverse American Anthropological Association (see above).

Brunel University
www.brunel.ac.uk/depts/hs/ MEDICANT.htm
A good website with information about the Msc in Medical Anthropology, the first taught Master's degree dedicated to Medical Anthropology in Europe. It is now not only one of the largest European social anthropology degrees, but has already produced 250 graduates.
Contact: Veronica Johnson, Human Sciences, Brunel University, Uxbridge, Middlesex, UB8 3PH (01895 274000 ext 3422.2452)

University College, London
http://www.ucl.ac.uk/Anthropology/index2
Another place where you can study medical anthropology.

The Royal Anthropological Institute (RAI)
www.therai.org.uk
The RAI is the world's longest-established scholarly association dedicated to the furtherance of anthropology (the study of humankind) in its broadest and most inclusive sense.

6 The range of clinical conditions in general practice

Surinder Singh, Joe Rosenthal, Jeannette Naish

What do we mean by clinical conditions? In its broadest sense, clinical care might be thought of as everything that goes on between health workers and patients. For the purpose of this chapter, however, we will use the term 'clinical' in a narrower sense that relates mainly to dealing with people who have 'illness'; although not so narrowly as to consider only those who have 'disease' (see Chapter 5). We do not attempt here to discuss in detail, or even list, the vast range of clinical conditions that can present in general practice. Instead, we aim to explore the general principles of clinical management using three examples from fairly distinct areas of practice. These cover different broad types of care: from episodic or acute care, in which the doctor addresses the problems of patients with acute episodes of illness (e.g. sore throat), through sub-acute care, as in the management of some sexually transmitted infections, to chronic care, as often takes place looking after elderly patients.

> **L** The MRCGP Examination Regulations contain guidance about the range of clinical conditions likely to be examined, as well as sample questions. A much more detailed version of the examination syllabus is in preparation as this book goes to press. It will be available with exam application packs from the RCGP or via its website: www.rcgp.org.uk

The distinction between acute and chronic conditions is, in reality, often blurred. Acute episodes of ill health for the patient could vary from short-lived, usually self-limiting common illnesses to acute exacerbations of a chronic condition and to serious medical emergencies. The way patients use words like 'acute', 'urgent' or 'chronic' is different from the way doctors use them and is more often related to severity of symptom than to its duration. The patient might also have different expectations of what can be done for the condition. This difference in understanding and perception of illness often results in the two parties having different agendas when they meet. This could have as much influence as the history, examination and investigation on the management of the problem.

Although the examples of clinical conditions used in this chapter are contrasting, several principles tie them together. The discussion does not aim to provide recipes for treating the conditions mentioned but rather to illustrate different points about them:

■ Common acute problems, such as sore throat, are not always straight-forward and might well involve complex considerations involving psychosocial issues and balancing evidence-based decision making with patient perspectives and expectations.

■ Although the wide remit of sexual health is not always in the forefront of GPs' minds, increasing awareness of the number of people who are at risk or actually suffering with sexual-health-related problems means that we will need to become more involved in the future.

■ The changing demography of the UK population means that care of the elderly is increasingly important and provides good illustration of how proactive management can earn dividends later on.

> **L** The principle of thinking laterally about everyday clinical presentations runs throughout the MRCGP exam, especially the written paper. Use the discussion of 'index conditions' in this chapter as a template for reflecting widely on how the care of common problems in a general practice setting differs from that in secondary care.

Acute care: sore throat

One of the problems with sore throat – irrespective of aetiology – is that psychosocial issues nearly always play a part in presentation, expectations or treatment. Although a clear history and examination are important, the decision will nearly always come down to whether an antibiotic is clinically indicated or not. Patient expectations are such that, in some cases, the inevitable happens and an antibiotic will be prescribed. Having said this, it is wise to be wary of the rarer causes of sore throat, which will need something other than a short discussion about antipyretics, lots of fluid, rest and 'Come and see me again if things are not improving'.

Sore throat has been chosen as an example of acute care because, although it is a very common symptom in general practice (with an estimated incidence of 75 cases per 1000 patients per year – the seventh most frequent condition seen by GPs) there is no standard advice about its management. It raises several questions as to how GPs manage acute self-limiting illness.

The main source of controversy in dealing with sore throat is when to treat with antibiotics. Bacteria are the causative organisms in less than 30% of sore throats presenting to GPs but studies in the late 1970s (Howie 1976, Howie & Hutchinson 1978, Howie et al 1971) showed that up to 75% of patients seen were prescribed an antibiotic. This percentage has probably reduced since the 1970s, but is still high.

There is no evidence that bacterial infections can be identified clinically and a throat swab cannot separate bacterial carrier state from pathological growth. Confirmation of infection requires a rise in the antistreptolysin-O (ASO) titre, the demonstration of which is not practical in the general practice situation, and it is still not clear if the rapid latex agglutination test for streptococcal antigen is a sensitive enough tool for use in practice.

So how are GPs deciding when to treat this condition with an antibiotic? If we consider this problem in the terms discussed above regarding factors that influence doctors' decisions, it seems likely that what probably happens is that we separate patients into two groups: those likely to benefit from antibiotics and those unlikely to benefit. We allocate to these groups on the basis of a clinical cluster of sore throat, high temperature, enlarged and tender tonsillar lymph nodes and pharyngeal exudate.

Perhaps the most important question is whether we are benefiting those patients for whom we do prescribe antibiotics. Do their symptoms resolve earlier? Are they protected from the potential complications of their possible streptococcal infection? Several studies suggest that the duration of the illness is not much affected by treatment. Whitfield & Hughes (1981) found no reduction in length of illness, irrespective of clinical findings of fever, lymphadenopathy or exudate. Brumfitt & Slater (1957), using parenteral penicillin, found duration shortened by just 24 h. As for prevention of sequelae, Howie and colleagues (1971, 1976, 1978) showed no reduction in suppurative complications, glomerulonephritis or rheumatic fever. More recently, systematic reviews have found a minimal effect of antibiotics in the treatment of sore throat, shortening symptoms by a duration of only about 8 h.

There is no doubt that another important influence on the decision to prescribe or not is the knowledge of psychosocial factors affecting the patient, for example, if he or she has an imminent examination or major social occasion to attend. Howie (1976) showed the same set of photographs of inflamed throats, but accompanied by different psychosocial background statements, to 634 doctors. It was found that psychosocial factors significantly altered the decision to treat in half the cases.

Pressures to prescribe can originate from:

- an urge to 'do something'
- a desire to demonstrate concern
- patient pressure and perhaps expectation
- fitting with partners' habits
- pressure from pharmaceutical companies
- an attempt to reduce consultation time
- medicolegal considerations
- knowledge of a placebo response (present in every 'drug')
- reducing likelihood of subsequent visit
- playing for time.

The decision about whether to prescribe for self-limiting illness is clearly not purely academic. Medication of any sort can produce side-effects, is expensive and might reduce patients' confidence in managing such illness themselves. Brooks (1987) describes three 'golden rules' that should be fulfilled in attempting to reduce the number of prescriptions given for such conditions:

1 You must really want to stop prescribing for acute self-limiting illness, and for reasons that are in the patient's best interest.
2 Your ideas and intentions must be communicated to your colleagues in the primary healthcare team because their behaviour can enhance or diminish your efforts.
3 If you do not offer the patient a prescription then that patient must leave the consulting room believing that he or she has obtained something more valuable.

- Sore throat occurs in 75 patients per 1000 per year
- Bacteria cause less than 30% of sore throats presenting to GPs
- Bacterial infection cannot be identified clinically
- Duration of sore throat is little affected by antibiotics
- Complications are not reduced by antibiotics
- Psychosocial factors are a major influence on prescribing
- Acute self-limiting illness can be managed sympathetically without writing a prescription

The purpose of discussing sore throat has been to illustrate that the management of an apparently straightforward problem in general practice is not a simple matter. The process of deciding on management depends not just on awareness of the currently accepted scientific knowledge but on a complex weighing-up of multiple factors operating in each individual case. You do need to keep up-to-date with developments across the board of clinical medicine, but that alone will not make you a 'good doctor'. You must also be aware of the many factors that influence your decision making and be skilled at discovering your patients' ideas about their problems. In areas of difficulty, do not be afraid to share your uncertainty with your patient and to negotiate a plan with him or her.

Other rarer causes of sore throat include:

- Epstein–Barr virus, glandular fever (how do you diagnose this?)
- Diphtheria (still fairly common in Eastern European countries)
- Vincent's angina
- (Peri-) tonsillar abscess
- Aphthous ulceration
- Sexually transmitted infections (see next section)
- Neoplasia.

L Note how so apparently routine a problem as 'sore throat' pulls together not just basic medical knowledge but also evidence-based medicine, the 'irrational' elements in prescribing, principles of health promotion and what Stott and Davis (1979) call 'modifying help-seeking behaviour'. Applying this breadth to your management of other common presentations will lift your performance in the written paper and orals and will make it much easier for you to find suitable cases for inclusion in your video submission.

Subacute care: sexually transmitted infections

This section will discuss sexually transmitted infections (STIs), HIV infection and AIDS. Due to lack of space, other blood-borne viral infections will be excluded, although some information appears on the websites listed at the end of the chapter.

It is useful to think about sexually transmitted infections in the following terms:

- prevention
- identification of people with STIs
- making a diagnosis
- treatment of STIs
- current hot topics in STIs.

Box 6.1
Trends in the UK's sexual health

■ There has been a dramatic rise in STIs in the UK since 1995. This is especially worrying because we are in the era of HIV/AIDS. Particular rises in infections occur in men who have sex with men, and also in teenage females.
■ Diagnoses of chlamydial infections have also risen sharply since the early 1990s (20% for men and 17% for women): this is partly due to increased awareness amongst the public, who now want to be tested. In 2001, genital chlamydial infection became the most common STI in England, Wales and Northern Ireland (see www.phls.co.uk).
■ There have been rises in major STIs such as gonorrhoea (increase of 31% in men and 26% in women).
■ There have been sporadic outbreaks of syphilis – in Cambridgeshire, London, Brighton and one or two other cities in the UK. These outbreaks have largely been in men who have sex with men.
■ Finally, while many of these statistics are worrying enough, they do not include diagnoses made in primary care. It is clear that, because a sizeable proportion of infections are diagnosed and treated in primary care, these figures are an underestimate (see www.phls.co.uk for further statistics).

Box 6.1 looks at some disturbing trends in sexually transmitted infections in the UK.

L   It is said that that the UK has some of the worst 'sexual health' in the developed world and certainly in Europe (only Ukraine is worse!). How do you think general practice – perhaps with an emphasis on its collaboration with public health – can contribute to reducing the morbidity associated with these rather depressing trends?

Prevention of STIs

In terms of STIs, primary prevention aims to stop the problem in the first place. Thus, using condoms, alerting people to the dangers of unsafe sex and acknowledging that multiple partners all increase risk of an STI are important. Secondary prevention aims to identify and, where possible, treat any condition before complications set in or symptomatic disease takes hold, for example by offering to take a chlamydia swab every time you see a woman who complains of a vaginal discharge. Tertiary prevention aims to manage the disease process. It is not uncommon in larger cities to see patients with previously identified HIV infection who receive no specialist input. So, whereas you, as the doctor, know that mortality and morbidity have fallen in the age of highly active antiretroviral therapy (HAART), the challenge is to communicate this to the patient who has chosen not to attend for specialist advice.

L For the exam, you need to be thoroughly familiar with the terminology, principles and practice of preventive interventions, particularly in such serious conditions as ischaemic heart disease, cerebrovascular disease and diabetes. See also Chapter 7.

Identification of individuals with STIs

How do you identify patients with STIs in the midst of a busy surgery? What are the barriers to doing this? And why do doctors still find it hard to take a comprehensive sexual history? There are several factors here and no single one accounts for all the reasons why taking a patient's sexual history does not occur as easily as, say, taking a cardiovascular history. The barriers are easy to identify, for example, taking a sexual history is sometimes embarrassing, the questions need to be very intimate and getting the words right can be difficult. Thus, taking a sexual history is delicate and often avoided. Like any skill, to gain confidence takes practice and role play with colleagues or actors is an excellent way to achieve this.

It is also clear that some infections, such as HIV and AIDS, are still highly stigmatised areas, which creates other problems. Confidentiality is also an issue, for example, patients might worry that if they tell you that they are gay then this information will get around to other members of staff, or even other people in the locality. Finally, identifying people with an STI requires a low level of suspicion and a desire to take a sensible, focused history.

Making a diagnosis

Making a diagnosis of an STI in primary care is no different from diagnosing any other condition. Thus, a thorough history, examination and investigations are the main methods. In terms of tests, the following can be useful:

- testing for common bacterial infections and viruses
- testing specifically for chlamydia infection – usually an endocervical swab
- blood sampling for syphilis where indicated
- blood sampling for viral infections, including HIV and hepatitis. It is always important to ensure that patient consent and confidentiality are discussed.

Primary presentation of STIs

- Vaginal or urethral discharge
- Dysuria and frequency
- Genital ulcers – painful or painless
- Testicular or epididymal pain in men
- A variety of rashes
- Lumps in genital/groin area

> **Secondary presentation of STIs**
>
> - Sterile pyuria
> - Pelvic pain and dyspareunia
> - Menstrual irregularities and breakthrough bleeding
> - Cervical smear abnormalities
> - Miscarriage
> - Ectopic pregnancy
> - Premature labour
> - Conjunctivitis
> - Reactive arthritis
> - Patient present with a 'contact slip'

In many ways, making a diagnosis is very much dependent on how much you want to make the diagnosis. Although many doctors prefer to send all patients to the local genitourinary (GU) clinic, for others, this aspect of their patients' care is no different to any other. With a good laboratory service and a basic understanding of microbiology and the presentation of sexual infections, much of STI diagnosis and management is possible in general practice.

Partner notification

It is sensible to know what the procedure is for partners, especially when you have identified something like chlamydia. What do you think you should do?

Partner notification means that you advise the patient to tell his or her partner(s) of the recently identified STI. Although this is a task previously always done by the GU clinic, the sheer numbers, and the fact that not everyone goes to a GU clinic, means that primary care often needs to take on this role as well. It is also appropriate for you to seek help in partner notification. Some practices are happy to proceed with a local protocol that identifies, treats and follows up patients with chlamydia but feel that partner notification is beyond their remit. This is fine so long as everyone agrees with this and you can be sure that all your patients will attend a GU clinic.

Partner notification is inevitably patient led. You can only go by what you have been told and, although it makes sense to encourage the 'index' patient to tell you about his or her partner(s) this will not always be possible, or the patient simply might not want to do this. The GU clinic often uses a formal procedure of giving out a partner notification contact slip, which is coded and merely asks the patient to attend any GU clinic anywhere in the country where their 'infection' will be treated. Once again, this is very much the domain of a specialist clinic and it is interesting that primary care does not have a similar system for this type of follow-up.

> **Other special features of STIs**
>
> ■ If you diagnose a sexually transmitted infection in a patient, test for others because there is a high probability of concurrent infections.
> ■ Remember partner notification. One of the reasons for the high rate of infection in the UK is poor notification of partner(s), which means that the overall pool of infection is high.
> ■ Where you don't know or are not sure about management – seek help. A friendly GU physician or senior clinical nurse specialist (CNS) in GU medicine are clinicians you can access without too much difficulty.
> ■ Please don't forget HIV infection. It is still the case that up to one-third of all people in the UK with HIV infection don't know about it. This is a great shame because there are now proven therapies that reduce morbidity and mortality.
> ■ Finally, remember that confidentiality and patient consent are fundamental to this aspect of care, as in any other. The fact that STIs are sensitive and sometimes stigmatising makes this even more of an issue.

Treatment of STIs

STIs come to light in primary care through normal surgeries and also through cervical smear programmes and family planning clinics. Although it is sensible to ensure good links with local GU services, some patients either don't want to go or choose not to be referred to the local clinic. It might therefore fall upon primary care to manage these problems.

There is a large body of opinion – amongst both GPs and GU specialists – that patients with a proven or suspected STI should always be referred to the local GU clinic for confirmation of diagnosis, treatment, counselling and the appropriate management of partner or partners. Although this might be true in an ideal world, we have to remember that only about half of people who are referred to GU clinics actually attend. This is a difficult dilemma but most clinicians would probably attempt to treat and strongly advise on partner notification where the patient refuses to attend the GU clinic. There might be local variations, depending on how accessible the GU clinic happens to be.

Current hot topics in STIs, including HIV infection and AIDS

The three specific areas chosen for this section represent developments in GU medicine that will impact on primary care, if not now, in the near future. These topics might well appear in any section of the MRCGP examination.

Chlamydial infection

There is debate as to whether chlamydial infection will ever be part of a systematic screening programme in the UK. What is clear, however, is that certain groups of people are at risk of infection:

- patients presenting with symptoms
- women seeking a termination of pregnancy
- asymptomatic sexually active women aged under 25 years, especially teenagers
- asymptomatic women aged over 25 years who have a new partner
- patients with another sexually transmitted infection.

This is an area of much development. In some pilot screening programmes, newer, more sensitive tests are being used. Women are advised how to take their own swabs and, for men, the advent of urine tests will almost certainly increase uptake of tests because it removes the need for the less acceptable urethral swab. The recently published National Strategy for sexual health and HIV implementation action plan announces that the next phase of chlamydia screening will take place at 10 different sites in England – this is something to be welcomed (for more details, see: www.doh.gov.uk/sexualhealthandhiv).

HIV and AIDS

Approximately 40 000 people are infected with HIV in the UK and unlinked anonymous surveys estimate that, in addition, about one-third of this number are unaware of being affected (DoH 2000). Of these infections, approximately three-quarters occur in gay men, and significant numbers in people from African communities and in injecting drug users. In 1999, for the first time there were more new infections with HIV than in previous years and transmission through heterosexual sex exceeded that through men having sex with men. There is no evidence to suggest any of this is changing.

Worryingly, transmission of HIV still occurs in gay men and bisexual men. Add to this the rising number of STIs in all groups and it is easy to see that unsafe sex is happening all the time. The prevalence of HIV continues to rise in pregnant women in both England and Scotland. A substantial proportion of infections occur in women born abroad – in the London area, 85% of women with HIV infection originate in sub-Saharan Africa. The Department of Health (DoH) established a target of an 80% diagnosis rate for pregnant women in inner London, which has been met. Nevertheless, the achievement of the national objective of an 80% reduction in mother-to-child transmission of HIV requires further improvement in the rate of antenatal HIV diagnosis outside London, as well as sustaining this improvement in London (DoH 2000).

Interventions that have proved effective in preventing vertical transmission of HIV

- Antiretroviral therapy before delivery for mother *and*
- Antiretroviral therapy for the newborn
- Delivery by elective caesarean section
- Avoiding breastfeeding

Despite this, there has been a substantial increase in the number of people diagnosed with HIV infection. In the UK between 1996 and 2002 there has been a 40% increase in the number of people with HIV infection, mainly due to the fall in mortality. There are still great regional variations in HIV prevalence. In Edinburgh, for example, the epidemic consists of people infected through sharing needles rather than through sexual transmission. Thus other blood-borne virus infections (hepatitis B and C) also continue to be a major problem. Although the degree of transmission through oral sex cannot be documented accurately it is now thought that the risk is higher than previously estimated (Hawkins 2001). It is now DoH policy to minimise this by recommending condoms for oral sex.

Treatment issues:
highly-active
antiretroviral
therapy (HAART)

One of the problems in HIV and AIDS is that, unlike the majority of other conditions, some patients will be suffering with chronic infection without their GP knowing about it. Despite this, the average London GP will know of patients on highly active antiretroviral therapy (HAART) and, increasingly, GPs outside London are also seeing patients on HAART regimes. It is difficult for GPs to keep up-to-date with the rapid developments in this field and good communication between specialist clinics and general practitioners is essential (Singh & Madge 1998, Singh et al 2001).

Chronic care:
health care for
older people

Caring for older people requires the integration of the many different skills of general practice, with input from community health and social care sectors. For the elderly, a holistic approach is especially critical; as well as providing medical care we must be aware of concerns regarding physical, psychological and social functioning. The proportion of the UK population over 75 is rising dramatically and this is reflected in the work of GPs in most areas. Many of the health problems of older people are the same as those that occur in the general adult population. There are, however, certain age-related needs that should be considered in their overall care (Illiffe & Drennan 2001). In 1990, the RCGP published an occasional paper entitled *Care of Old People* (Baker 1990), which offers a useful framework for looking after older people in general practice. A 12-point list of objectives in the care of older people is outlined:

1 To maintain and, where possible, improve the quality of life for elderly people by a regular programme of medical audit.
2 To keep abreast of new developments in health care by a commitment to continuing medical education.
3 To take into account old people's problems in gaining access to the available services provided by the practice.
4 To strive to reach accurate diagnoses on which logical treatment and realistic progress can be based.

5 To provide effective continuing care for those with long-term medical problems and chronic illness.

6 To offer a systematic programme of anticipatory health care for older people.

7 To contribute to the resettlement of patients who are discharged from hospital or other institutions back into the community.

8 To provide sensitive and effective care for the dying patient.

9 To develop and participate in a team approach to the provision of the care of elderly persons.

10 To provide information and health education to older people in the practice.

11 To support the informal carers with the aim of preventing breakdown.

12 To further the interests of older people and, when necessary, act as their advocate.

The National Service Framework for Older People

The Department of Health published a National Service Framework (NSF) for Older People in 1999 (Box 6.2; see also Chapter 7). This was developed with the advice of an External Reference Group, which brought together expert input from older people and their carers, healthcare and social care professionals, managers and partner agencies in the voluntary sector. National standards of care were set to ensure:

- high-quality care and treatment, regardless of age
- that older people are treated as individuals, with respect and dignity
- fair resources for the conditions that most affect older people
- easing of the financial burden of long-term residential care.

Embedded in the standards are the declared NHS core principles that services should reach those most in need and that there should be equity in access to services for all older people.

Medical care

The medical part of continuing care concerns monitoring the effects of treatment, how the patient is progressing and, most importantly, the early diagnosis and prevention of the complications of disease (tertiary prevention). Older people can suffer from several complex interacting conditions all at the same time. Medical management therefore needs to be tailored accordingly. This involves regular review and a systematic examination of patients on long-term medication. The hazards of prescribing for patients with compromised renal and liver functions, using multiple medicines, are well known. Care needs to be taken, with the doctor constantly alert to drug interactions and complications. Here, the local pharmacist could be an invaluable resource. The use of clinical protocols is often advocated. The process of writing a protocol should allow the doctor(s) to consider what constitutes good clinical practice in the management of a particular chronic condition.

Box 6.2
The eight National Service Framework standards for older people (NHSE 1999)

Standard one: rooting out age discrimination
NHS services will be provided, regardless of age, on the basis of clinical need alone. Social Care services will not use age in their eligibility criteria or policies, to restrict access to available services.

Standard two: person-centred care
NHS and Social Care services treat older people as individuals and enable them to make choices about their own care. This is achieved through the single assessment process, integrated commissioning arrangements and integrated provision of services, including community equipment and continence services.

Standard three: intermediate care
Older people will have access to a new range of intermediate care services at home or in designated care settings to promote their independence by providing enhanced services from the NHS and councils to prevent unnecessary hospital admission and effective rehabilitation services to enable early discharge from hospital and to prevent premature or unnecessary admission to long-term residential care.

Standard four: general hospital care
Older people's care in hospital is delivered through appropriate specialist care and by hospital staff who have the right set of skills to meet their needs.

Standard five: stroke
The NHS will take action to prevent strokes, working in partnership with other agencies where appropriate.
People who are thought to have had a stroke have access to diagnostic services, are treated appropriately by a specialist stroke service and, subsequently, with their carers, participate in a multidisciplinary programme of secondary prevention and rehabilitation.

Standard six: falls
The NHS, working in partnership with councils, takes action to prevent falls and reduce resultant fractures or other injuries in their populations of older people.
Older people who have fallen receive effective treatment and rehabilitation and, with their carers, receive advice on prevention through a specialised falls service.

Standard seven: mental health in older people
Older people who have mental health problems have access to integrated mental health services, provided by the NHS and councils to ensure effective diagnosis, treatment and support, for them and for their carers.

Standard eight: promoting an active healthy life in older age
The health and well-being of older people is promoted through a coordinated programme of action led by the NHS with support from councils.

Social support

Empathy, compassion and continuity of care are important to patients and carers. Seeing a patient regularly, especially when it requires a home visit, may not seem to be an efficient use of time in the medical sense but it could mean a lot to the patient and carers as an expression of interest and concern, and provide a source of emotional support. At the same time, it gives an opportunity to identify possible risk factors in vulnerable people, which in turn allows preventative action to be taken. This principle holds for all health professionals caring for older people, where integrated, multiprofessional input is essential. The aim would be to maintain independent functioning as far as possible. A case study of a hospital discharge would illustrate the processes of assessing the need for services required to maintain independent living, not forgetting welfare rights and benefits. Many older people miss out on their entitlement to benefits, often through a lack of information.

Time constraints mean that most GPs have to be selective about visiting chronically ill people at home. In general, a person with good social support would be less likely to be on the chronic visiting list, especially if visits to the surgery are appropriate, whereas isolated, housebound older people living alone might value a visit from their doctor, despite attention from district nurses and social service home care teams.

Most, if not all, GPs give supportive psychotherapy, sometimes without knowing. Michael Balint (1957) was the first to describe this phenomenon. If the role of the GP as a generalist is to be preserved then this supportive role must remain. Medical education and hospital practice tend to emphasise the 'medical model' of diagnosis, investigation and surgical or medical treatment (see Chapter 5). The idea of maintaining quality of life is perhaps given more priority in general practice, where people are seen more in their own surroundings. The social and supportive role of the doctor and the value of a relationship built up over many years might not be measurable, nor fall neatly into a box for ticking in a management protocol.

Case study
Mr G, who lives alone

Mr G has recently celebrated his eighty-fourth birthday. He has lived alone in his second-floor, one-bedroom flat since his wife died 5 years ago. There is no lift. His only daughter is married with three teenaged children; the youngest has just turned thirteen. She loves her Dad, and visits at least once every fortnight (she lives several hundred miles away); they talk on the telephone almost every day.

Although managing well on his own, Mr G has suffered with high blood pressure for many years. He developed angina soon after his wife died. He takes his blood pressure and heart tablets as ordered by the doctor but has recently had difficulty managing the stairs because of arthritis in both knees, and cannot go out much, even to get his pension or his shopping, without a neighbour's help. He was prescribed 'arthritis' tablets by the GP. He has noticed that he cannot walk more than 20 yards on the flat without getting pain in his calves. He also noticed that his ankles have been swelling slightly since he started on the 'arthritis' tablets.

Mr G doesn't bother the doctor much, except to get repeat prescriptions, but he woke up one night very short of breath. He had to sit up most of the night and was so frightened that he asked the doctor to visit first thing.

You find that Mr G is in mild congestive cardiac failure. You believe that with effective monitoring by a district nurse, and with home care support, you could get the failure under control at home. You are, however, aware that although the district nurse could visit, this would not be more than once a day, and only for a day or two because of staff shortages. Social services would not be able to do an assessment for at least a week. Under these circumstances, you feel that Mr G should be admitted to hospital. Mr G refuses to go.

The following are issues that you may like to consider:

- What are the practical and ethical issues at the point when you suggest hospital admission?
- Would admitting Mr G be an 'unnecessary' hospital admission, as formulated in the NSF for older people?
- On reflection, how would you manage Mr G's medication?
- If Mr G agreed to hospital admission, what services would be needed (in an ideal world) to support him for independent living in his own home on discharge?
- Could the level of support for Mr G to return to his flat be available or sustainable in your locality? If not, what are the ethical dilemmas relating to the allocation of community services for people who are highly dependent but wish to live at home?
- Should Mr G be persuaded to go into a residential home?
- What might have been done to prevent this crisis?

Conclusions

This chapter set out to examine the range of clinical conditions encountered in general practice. We have discussed examples aiming to cover acute, subacute and chronic problems and hope that this has illustrated not only the variety of clinical work involved in general practice but also the fact that, to provide a modern primary healthcare service we must do much more than provide reactive 'medical care' for individual patients as they present with their problems. We must be able to consider changes in population need, to predict and assess individual patients' needs on several different levels and to work with colleagues from different disciplines to meet those needs. These diverse conditions contribute to both the challenge and the reward of a career in general practice.

Summary

■ The ideas of tertiary prevention are central to caring for older people.

■ The main aim of care of older people is not 'cure' or improvement in the disease but the alleviation of suffering and the maintenance or improvement of the levels of functioning and quality of life.

■ Established disease needs to be recognised early, whether during chronic disease monitoring or active screening.

■ Social support or treatment should be initiated to minimise possible functional impairment caused by illness and to improve the quality of life.

References

Baker R 1990 Care of old people; a framework for progress. RCGP Occasional Paper no. 45. RCGP, London

Balint M 1957 The doctor, his patient and the illness, 2nd edn. Churchill Livingstone, Edinburgh

Brooks D 1987 How to stop prescribing for acute self-limiting conditions. Update 15 August 1987: 311–317

Brumfitt W, Slater JDM 1957 Treatment of acute sore throat with penicillin. Lancet 1:8–11

DoH 2000 Prevalence of HIV and hepatitis infections in the UK. Unlinked Anonymous Prevalence Monitoring Programme in the United Kingdom. Public Health Laboratory Services/Department of Health, London. Online. Available: http://www.doh.gov.uk

Hawkins S 2001 Oral sex and HIV transmission. Sexually Transmitted Infections 77:307–308

Howie JGR 1976 Clinical judgement and antibiotic use in general practice. British Medical Journal 2:1061–1064

Howie JGR, Hutchinson KR 1978 Antibiotics and respiratory illness in general practice; prescribing policy and workload. British Medical Journal 2:1342

Howie JGR, Richardson IM, Gill D, Durno D 1971 Respiratory illness and antibiotic use in general practice. Journal of the Royal College of General Practitioners 21:657–663

Illiffe S, Drennan V 2001 Primary care for older people. Oxford University Press, Oxford

National Health Service Executive (NHSE) 1999 National Service Framework for Older People. Department of Health, London

Singh S, Madge S 1998 The general practitioner and the primary health care team. In: Singh S, Madge S (eds) Caring for people with HIV infection and AIDS. Ashgate Publishing, Aldershot, pp 93–106

Singh S, Carter Y, Dunford A 2001 Routine care of people with HIV infection and AIDS: should interested general practitioners take the lead? British Journal of General Practice 51:399–403

Stott NCH, Davis RH 1979 The exceptional potential in each primary care consultation. Journal of the Royal College of General Practitioners 29:201–205

Whitfield MJ, Hughes AO 1981 Penicillin in acute sore throat. Practitioner 225:234–239

Further reading

Department of Health 2001 National sexual health strategy. Online. Available: www.doh.gov.uk/nshs/summary.htm

Sexually transmitted infections. Report from BMA Board of Science and Education. Online. February 200

Useful sexual health/HIV and AIDS care websites for health professionals

www.agum.org.uk
Information from the Association of Genitourinary Medicine, useful information for specialists and contains information about clinical effectiveness guidelines.

www.avert.org.uk/about.htm
An example of a leading UK charity focused on UK AIDS education and research. Particularly useful for a range of school education around HIV and AIDS.

www.bma.org.uk
British Medical Association website. See the Report from the BMA Board of Science and Education entitled Sexually transmitted infections.

www.doh.gov.uk/nshs/summary.htm
The website for the Department of Health National Sexual Health Strategy.

www.fertilityuk.org
Website for fertility awareness and natural family planning.

www.fpa.org.uk
More related to the fields of contraception and sexual health. This website is for both professionals and the public.

www.margaretpyke.org
Website for the Margaret Pyke Centre in London.

www.medfash.org.uk
Website for the Medical Foundation for AIDS and Sexual Health, a charity that works with health professionals to meet the challenges of HIV and other sexually transmitted infections. The work centres on influencing policy and providing information and advice to professionals.

www.mssvd.org.uk
Again, an example of a specialist website that attempts to educate all about sexually transmitted infections and sexual health in general.

www.nat.org.uk
The umbrella organisation of leading partnerships to fight HIV infection and AIDS in the UK.

www.phls.co.uk/facts/index.htm
An absolutely excellent website for those interested in public health issues. It contains a list of facts and figures about many conditions. The ready-made slide show is recommended.

www.phls.co.uk/publications/CDR
Communicable diseases review is an information sheet, now produced electronically, which highlights general news on infections, outbreaks and their subsequent investigation.

www.tht.org.uk
Perhaps the leading UK-based HIV/AIDS charity with specialist advisors who can help on various issues related to HIV and AIDS. Also now includes what used to be London Lighthouse.

Useful websites for patients, including for adolescents/a young audience

www.avert.org/yngindx.htm
A site containing information for young people and particularly for young gay men. Also contains information about puberty, contraception and HIV/AIDS.

www.brook.org.uk
Again, a site for young people. Contains FAQs designed specifically for the 16–25-year-old group. This will also direct you to the many clinics (with maps) in the inner cities.

www.likeitis.org.uk
Young people's site set up by Marie Stopes International.

www.llgs.org.uk
Website for London Lesbian and Gay Switchboard.

www.playingsafely.co.uk
Another site for youngsters containing a welter of information on sex, HIV, contraception, including how to use a condom properly and what safer sex really is.

www.ruthinking.co.uk
Website for the under-18s. It supports the sex-wise campaign, which is a free confidential help-line for people wanting to know about relationships, sex and contraception.

7 Promoting health, preventing disease

Joe Rosenthal, Margaret Lloyd

In the early stages of medical training, most of us are keener to learn about diagnosing and managing disease than preventing disease and promoting health. However, as we develop into independent practitioners and see for ourselves the prevalence and the cost of preventable health problems, we realise that prevention really is better than cure. The GP's responsibility is to care for both the individual patient and the whole practice population. Prevention strategies should therefore be aimed at both the individual, particularly those at high risk, and the practice population.

This chapter will examine the scope in general practice for preventing disease and promoting health, the underlying principles involved and how best we can approach the challenge. This is a lot to cover in one chapter and we cannot provide a comprehensive account of all the preventive activities carried out in general practice. The aim therefore is to help the registrar to think critically about what is, and what can be, done in the context of prevention in general practice.

We will deal first with some basic definitions then go on to examine the opportunities for prevention in general practice, the roles of government and the primary healthcare team, and finally the theoretical concepts underlying screening and health education activities.

Definition of terms in prevention

Several related terms are used and often confused in discussions of prevention. These are: 'health promotion', 'primary', 'secondary' and 'tertiary prevention', 'health education', 'health protection'. In a nutshell, health promotion emphasises the dual role of preventing ill health and promoting positive health. The primary healthcare team is predominantly involved in prevention and health education. Health protection activities lie more in the public health domain.

Health promotion

Health promotion has been defined as 'the efforts to enhance positive health and prevent ill-health through the overlapping spheres of health education, prevention and health protection' (Downie et al 1990).

Prevention

Prevention is about reducing the risk of a disease process, illness, injury or disability. It includes preventive services (e.g. immunisation and screening), preventive health education (e.g. advice about sensible drinking) and preventive health protection (e.g. taxing tobacco and fluoridating water). Preventive activities are often classified as primary, secondary or tertiary prevention. These reflect the stages in the natural history of the disease at which the intervention is made.

Primary prevention includes all activities that remove the cause of disease or decrease the susceptibility of the individual to the causative agent. Many primary preventive activities should be part of the national strategy. In general practice, examples of primary prevention include:

- health education, e.g. advice about smoking
- immunisation.

Secondary prevention is synonymous with screening and describes the detection and treatment of disease before symptoms or disordered function develops, that is, before irreversible damage occurs. Examples include:

- cervical screening
- screening for hypertension.

Tertiary prevention is the monitoring and management of established disease to prevent disability or handicap. An example is:

■ monitoring of patients with diabetes to detect and treat early complications.

This classification has been criticised on the grounds that it focuses on disease and includes treatment, and that there is no standard definition of the terms primary, secondary and tertiary. For example, the term 'secondary prevention' is sometimes used to describe interventions that aim to prevent recurrence of an illness (e.g. the use of aspirin after myocardial infarction). All classifications draw boundaries that at times seem artificial, but these are useful as long as the reservations are borne in mind and the classification of prevention is no exception to this.

Health education

Health education aims to diminish ill health and enhance positive health by influencing people's beliefs, attitudes and behaviour. A central theme is helping (or empowering) individuals to build on their assets and to make appropriate choices for healthy living. This will be discussed in greater detail later in this chapter.

Health protection

Health protection activities are usually public health measures and include legal and fiscal controls and other regulations laid down by government. These measures increase the chance of people living in a healthy environment and should help to make healthy choices easier choices.

Opportunities for prevention in general practice

The opportunities for disease prevention and health promotion in general practice are diverse; the most important are listed in Box 7.1.

Box 7.1
Opportunities for prevention in general practice

Antenatal/children
Antenatal care, smoking/alcohol in pregnancy, developmental screening, routine immunisations, accidents

Adolescence
Contraception, safer sex, smoking, alcohol, drugs, rubella immunisation

Adults
Smoking, alcohol, diet, exercise, contraception, safer sex, breast screening, cervical screening, blood pressure screening, immunisation boosters

Elderly
Screening for functional problems, tetanus immunisation, influenza immunisation

The scope for prevention

Where should efforts to prevent ill health be directed? One approach is to look at the major causes of mortality and morbidity in the population today. At the beginning of the twentieth century, 40% of all deaths were due to infectious diseases. Now these account for a very small proportion of total deaths. Cancer, ischaemic heart disease, cerebrovascular disease and accidents have become the major causes of premature death (i.e. death before the age of 64 years) and total mortality.

Many of the risk factors associated with cancer and cardiovascular disease have been identified and are potentially modifiable. But prevention is not only about prolonging life, it is also about reducing morbidity, enabling people to lead fulfilling lives for as long as possible.

> **L** Governments are often thought to shirk health promotion measures that appear to lie within their power, e.g. by banning tobacco advertising or imposing stricter drink-driving legislation. What should be the response of GPs, individually and collectively, in the face of such apparent failure of the State to take responsibility?

The role of the government in prevention

Government policies and national strategies play a fundamental role in prevention. For example, during the nineteenth century mortality from tuberculosis was falling long before the tubercle bacillus was identified and chemotherapy was developed, largely because of the improvement in nutrition and living conditions related to social and political change.

Strategies aimed at preventing ill health should operate on at least four levels. For example, an effective programme to reduce alcohol-related problems and deaths might involve:

- *Government and national strategies*:
  - increased taxation on alcohol
  - advertising restrictions
  - changes in the law concerning drinking and driving.
- *District strategies*:
  - local health education programme about sensible drinking in schools and workplaces.
- *Practice strategies*:
  - increased efforts to identify and help individuals who are drinking at hazardous levels.
- *Individual strategies*:
  - each individual to review his or her alcohol consumption and to decide (with help if necessary) if they need to modify it.

> **L** Questions about screening are a very popular topic of discussion in the MRCGP oral exam. Many suggestions are made in the medical or popular press for possible screening programmes, e.g. for bowel or testicular cancer. You should be able readily to appraise such proposals in the light of 'Wilson's criteria' (see p. 97).

Box 7.2
*Health of the Nation
1992 – key areas for
action*

- Coronary heart disease and stroke
- Cancers
- Mental illness
- HIV/AIDS and sexual health
- Accidents

In 1992, the Department of Health published a White Paper entitled *The Health of the Nation* (Secretary of State for Health 1992). This set out a strategy for improving the health of the population of England by identifying key areas for action, setting targets for reducing incidence in each area and suggesting strategies for achieving them within a defined period of time (Box 7.2).

This approach of setting priorities and targets for prevention has subsequently been developed within the system, introduced by the present Labour Government, of National Service Frameworks (NSFs).

*National Service
Frameworks*

Papers produced by the Labour Government, including *The NHS Plan* (Secretary of State for Health 2000), *The New NHS* (Secretary of State for Health 1997) and *A First Class Service* (Secretary of State for Health 1998) (all available via the NHS publications website: www.doh.gov.uk/help/publications.htm) introduced a range of measures to raise quality and decrease variations in service. One of these measures was the introduction of National Service Frameworks (NSFs). These frameworks aim to:

- set national standards and define service models for a defined service or care group
- put in place strategies to support implementation
- establish performance milestones against which progress within an agreed time-scale will be measured.

The rolling programme of NSFs was launched in April 1998. At the time of writing, NSFs have been published for mental health, coronary heart disease (CHD), and care of older people. Related to the NSF programme, a National Cancer Plan was published in September 2000. Development is underway for frameworks to follow in diabetes, renal services, children's services, and long-term conditions focusing on neurological problems. Full details of the existing NSFs, and plans for forthcoming frameworks, can be found on the Department of Health website (www.doh.gov/nsf).

Each NSF is developed with the assistance of an External Reference Group (ERG), which brings together health professionals, service users and carers, health service managers, partner agencies and other advocates. The Department of Health supports the ERGs and manages the overall process. Although the name and aims of the NSFs puts emphasis on service, there is no doubt that all the NSFs will include measures targeted at primary, secondary and tertiary prevention. An example of this can be seen in the Coronary Heart Disease NSF standards (Table 7.1).

Table 7.1 *Standards table from Coronary Heart Disease National Service Framework*

Standard	Actions
Standards 1 and 2: reducing heart disease in the population	1 *The NHS and partner agencies* should develop, implement and monitor policies that reduce the prevalence of coronary risk factors in the population, and reduce inequalities in risks of developing heart disease 2 *The NHS and partner agencies* should contribute to a reduction in the prevalence of smoking in the local population
Standards 3 and 4: preventing CHD in high-risk patients	3 *General practitioners and primary healthcare teams* should identify all people with established cardiovascular disease and offer them comprehensive advice and appropriate treatment to reduce their risks 4 *General practitioners and primary healthcare teams* should identify all people at significant risk of cardiovascular disease but who have not developed symptoms and offer them appropriate advice and treatment to reduce their risks
Standards 5, 6 and 7: heart attack and other acute coronary syndromes	5 *People with symptoms of a possible heart attack* should receive help from an individual equipped with and appropriately trained in the use of a defibrillator within 8 min of calling for help, to maximise the benefits of resuscitation should it be necessary 6 *People thought to be suffering from a heart attack* should be assessed professionally and, if indicated, receive aspirin. Thrombolysis should be given within 60 min of calling for professional help 7 *NHS Trusts* should put in place agreed protocols/systems of care so that people admitted to hospital with proven heart attack are appropriately assessed and offered treatments of proven clinical and cost effectiveness to reduce their risk of disability and death
Standard 8: stable angina	8 *People with symptoms of angina or suspected angina* should receive appropriate investigation and treatment to relieve their pain and reduce their risk of coronary events
Standards 9 and 10: revascularisation	9 *People with angina that is increasing in frequency or severity* should be referred to a cardiologist urgently or, for those at greatest risk, as an emergency 10 *NHS Trusts* should put in place hospital-wide systems of care so that patients with suspected or confirmed coronary heart disease receive timely and appropriate investigation and treatment to relieve their symptoms and reduce their risk of subsequent coronary events
Standard 11: heart failure	11 *Doctors* should arrange for people with suspected heart failure to be offered appropriate investigations (e.g. electrocardiography, echocardiography) that will confirm or refute the diagnosis. For those in whom heart failure is confirmed, its cause should be identified – treatments most likely to both relieve their symptoms and reduce their risk of death should be offered
Standard 12: cardiac rehabilitation	12 *NHS Trusts* should put in place agreed protocols/systems of care so that, prior to leaving hospital, people admitted to hospital suffering from coronary heart disease have been invited to participate in a multidisciplinary programme of secondary prevention and cardiac rehabilitation. The aim of the programme will be to reduce their risk of subsequent cardiac problems and to promote their return to a full and normal life

The effect of these NSFs on workload in primary care should not be underestimated. For example, the requirement just to collect and share data in the Coronary Heart Disease NSF is daunting. The RCGP has pointed out that, given that an average general practice consultation lasts between 7 and 10 min, one additional minute spent entering data after a consultation could have the effect of increasing general practitioner workload by between 10 and 15%. The answer is likely to lie in sharing the additional tasks involved in achieving NSF standards with other staff, who will need to be trained and paid to take on these additional duties.

The role of the primary healthcare team in prevention

The primary healthcare team has a unique role to play in the prevention of disease and the promotion of health. In the past, the job of the GP was seen mainly in terms of responding to individuals who presented their problems to her or him. Diagnosis and management were the doctor's main activities, and prevention of disease was not a high priority.

A move towards more proactive GP work gathered momentum in the 1970s, steered by reports from both the government and the RCGP, which stressed the importance of anticipatory care, that is, anticipating people's problems and trying to prevent them from happening. Anticipatory care implies the union of prevention with care and cure. Care of the individual patient presenting with, for example, an upper respiratory tract infection, should include appropriate preventive activity, e.g. blood pressure screening.

In 1990 the requirement for 'advice on general health and consultations and examinations to prevent disease' became, for the first time, part of the GP's terms of service. In addition, the government at that time provided extra funds for health promotion in practices. Prevention of disease and promotion of health, for which specific skills and training are necessary, have since become firmly established as a central part of the work of the GP and the primary healthcare team. It is already clear that significant emphasis is placed on this work in personal medical services (PMS) contracts and in the preliminary proposals for the new GP contract (see Chapter 16).

Strategies for prevention

There are two possible strategies for disease prevention and health promotion. The population strategy aims to reduce the risk of the whole population, usually by public health measures. The high-risk strategy focuses on the individual who is considered to be at high risk.

The rationale behind the population strategy is that the bulk of the morbidity and mortality of a disease in a population is contributed by those who have a moderate degree of risk. For example, the British Regional Heart Study found that 60% of middle-aged British men have total cholesterol (TC) levels that carry at least a twofold risk of major CHD; one-third of all heart attacks occur in the 20% of men with the highest levels of TC. The most effective way of reducing morbidity and mortality from CHD would be to move the population mean cholesterol level to the left, thus reducing the risk of the majority. In the case of cholesterol, this would be mainly by dietary means (i.e. reducing the proportion of calories from saturated fat). This is most likely to be achieved by public health measures, for example, general health education, food and pricing policy, labelling of foods and so on.

Another example of a population strategy is the reduction of alcohol-related morbidity and mortality. Reducing the number of people drinking at moderate risk levels (14–35 units/week in women and 21–50 units in men) would have a greater effect than identifying and offering treatment to those drinking at harmful levels (>35 units for women, >50 units for men).

Although public health measures (e.g. dietary recommendations, raising the taxes on cigarettes and alcohol) are the most effective population strategies at a national level, the population strategy also has a part to play in prevention at a practice level. For example, it is appropriate to give everybody in a practice dietary advice aimed at reducing serum cholesterol, as it can be safely assumed that everybody has a level that carries some risk of coronary heart disease.

The high-risk individual approach comes more naturally to the clinician. This approach aims to identify and treat individuals with a high risk of developing a disease (e.g. those with familial hypercholesterolaemia, individuals with high alcohol consumption). A combination of these two approaches is desirable in a general practice (i.e. dietary advice to everybody in the practice with screening and, when indicated, specific treatment, perhaps with lipid-lowering drugs, of those at particularly high risk).

Screening

A wide range of screening procedures are carried out in general practice (Box 7.3). The possibility of being able to detect and treat presymptomatic

Box 7.3
Screening procedures in general practice

Antenatal screening
Down syndrome, neural tube defects, syphilis, rubella

Neonatal
Phenylketonuria, congenital hypothyroidism, congenital dislocation of the hip, undescended testes, heart disease, developmental disorders

Childhood
Immunisation status, visual/hearing impairment, mental and physical development

Adults
Risk factors for coronary heart disease and stroke, cigarette smoking, alcohol consumption, blood cholesterol level, blood pressure, weight, cervical cancer, breast cancer

Old age
Sight and hearing, mobility, mental state, anaemia, blood pressure

disease, and to prevent or at least reduce its morbidity and mortality, seems desirable. The finding of hidden morbidity amongst the people screened, for example at the pioneer health centre at Peckham in the 1920s, and the description by Last (1963) of the 'iceberg of disease', provided the impetus to an expansion of screening activities. However, not all conditions are amenable to screening and the costs and benefits must be weighed up carefully before any screening programme is implemented. The idea of a periodic 'general check-up' has some logical appeal but research, such as that of the South East London Screening Study Group (1977), has found little evidence for the benefit of multiphasic screening of asymtomatic patients in terms of the time spent in detecting only a very few treatable abnormalities. Most effort with respect to screening has therefore focused on specific, common, serious and treatable conditions.

What is screening?

Screening is synonymous with secondary prevention and can be defined as the questioning, examination or investigation of an asymptomatic individual to determine the presence or absence of disease. A screening test is not intended to be diagnostic. It is used to distinguish apparently well persons who appear to have the disease that is being screened for from those who probably do not have the disease.

Various screening strategies have been described and the terminologies can be confusing. Some commonly used definitions are:

- *Population* or *mass screening* – a screening procedure that is offered to a whole population.
- *Multiple* or *multiphasic screening* – when a variety of screening tests are carried out at the same time. This type of screening is often adopted by the private health care organisations offering screening packages.
- *Selective screening* – the offering of a screening procedure to selected groups in a population that are considered to have an increased risk of having the condition, for example, mammography for women aged over 50 years.
- *Surveillance* – the long-term observation of individuals or population, for example, developmental screening for preschool children.
- *Case finding* – the screening of patients already in contact with the health services and the same as opportunistic screening. The contact, but not always the screening activity, is usually patient initiated.

Important characteristics of all types of screening are that the person being screened is asymptomatic for the condition being sought and that the intervention is usually initiated by the doctor. Ideally, the person or team responsible for the care of the individual should carry out the screening procedure. Any intervention or treatment that is required is then an integral part of the individual's overall care. Screening carried out by a group or organisation that does not have responsibility of the overall care of the individual is an example of the separation of prevention from care and cure.

Why carry out screening?

The majority of screening procedures carried out in general practice aim to improve the health and life expectancy of the individual patient. The term 'prescriptive screening' is often used in this context. Screening might be carried out in the interest of people other than the patient. The best example of this is screening of contacts of a patient found to have tuberculosis. Pre-employment screening and routine examinations for insurance purposes were the earliest examples of screening.

What conditions should be screened for?

L Despite the merits extolled in this chapter, health education fails to enthuse significant numbers of GPs. Why is this? What additional skills might be needed, or attitudes changed, to make these GPs more effective? How might the skills of professional educators, such as teachers or health visitors, be better harnessed?

The criteria that should be fulfilled before screening for a particular condition is adopted were defined by Wilson and Jungner (quoted in Holland & Stewart 1990) and are given below:

1 The condition should be an *important health problem.*
2 The *natural history* of the disease should be adequately understood.
3 There should be a *recognisable latent* or *early symptomatic stage.*
4 There should be a *suitable test* or *examination*, that is, the test is simple to perform and interpret, acceptable to those taking part, accurate and repeatable, and sensitive and specific.
5 Treatment started at an early stage should be of more benefit than treatment started at a later stage.
6 There should be *accepted treatment* for patients with recognised disease.
7 There should be an agreed policy on who should receive treatment.
8 Diagnosis and treatment should be cost effective.
9 Case finding should be a continuing process.

Screening test characteristics

Ideally, a screening test should select only those people who, on further testing, are found to have the disease (i.e. it should have 100% sensitivity). All people without the disease should produce a negative screening test (i.e. the test should be 100% specific). In reality, the ideal test does not exist, as we shall see by considering the specificity, sensitivity and predictive power of a screening test in greater detail.

The sensitivity of a screening test is the ability of a test to identify correctly those individuals who have the disease, as determined by a reference test (e.g. histological confirmation). It is a measure of the true positive rate. A highly sensitive test will have a low false negative rate. Ultrasound scanning for ovarian cancer is, for example, problematic as a single screening test because it has low sensitivity (i.e. there is a significant chance that small tumours will be missed).

The specificity of a screening test is the ability of the test to identify correctly those who do not have the disease. It is a measure of the true negative rate. A highly specific test will have a low false positive rate. Prostatic-specific antigen (PSA) testing for prostate carcinoma is, for example, problematic as a screening test because it has low specificity (i.e. several other reasons, apart from prostate cancer, can cause a raised PSA level).

The other important characteristics of a test are its positive and negative predictive values:

- The positive predictive value is the proportion of patients with a positive screening test who actually have the disease.
- The negative predictive value is the proportion of patients who screen negative who do not have the disease.

It is important to understand that the predictive value of a test depends on the prevalence of the disease (i.e. the total number of cases in a population) that is being screened for. If a disease is common in the population that is being screened, then the proportion of true positives is greater than when the prevalence is low.

Health education

One of the most important roles of the primary healthcare team is as educators, providing patients with information and support to enable them to make appropriate choices for healthy living. Other agencies are involved in health education, including government, schools, local health promotion units and the media. In general practice, health education activities must reinforce the work of these other agencies. The areas in which health education is most likely to be given in general practice are:

- helping patients to avoid disease and to promote their well-being, for example by providing advice on diet, sensible drinking and how to stop smoking
- helping patients to understand the importance of taking up the offer of screening procedures
- helping patients who have established disease to adopt behaviours that reduce disability
- educating patients about the appropriate use of health service resources.

Approaches to health education

Three approaches to health education are often described:

1 disease-oriented
2 risk-factor-oriented
3 health-oriented.

In disease-oriented health education there is a focus on a particular disease (e.g. cardiovascular disease) and the action is focused on the risk factors (e.g. providing dietary advice). The problem with this approach is that there is an overlap in risk factors for many types of disease (e.g. smoking for coronary heart disease and lung cancer), and the orientation is expert dominated, with the expert (the doctor) focusing on an area of his or her expertise (disease) and imparting information to the patient. The focus is a negative one, emphasising prevention of disease rather than promotion of health.

An alternative approach is to focus attention and action on risk factors rather than on the associated disease (e.g. focusing on smoking as a risk factor for carcinoma of the lung and coronary heart disease). This process recognises that single risk factors can be linked to more than one disease and therefore there is less duplication. However, the approach is still expert dominated and the emphasis is again on disease prevention rather than health promotion.

The health-oriented approach focuses attention and action on behaviour that contributes to positive health and prevents ill health. For example, it can be pointed out that a healthy diet can be enjoyable, contributing to well-being in a positive way rather than just being a way of preventing diseases.

Health education is about helping individuals to adopt behaviours that promote health. We must remember that the decision to change belongs to the patient and that his or her ability to change depends not only on motivation and individual skills, but also on the environment. However well motivated an individual is, it is undoubtedly more difficult to follow a healthy lifestyle on an inadequate income, in bad housing and if working in a dangerous environment. In providing health education we are aiming to help people to take control over decisions that affect their health, not simply providing information and expecting a change in behaviour.

Health education in practice

Health education involves exchanging (not just giving) information. This means that there must be good and effective channels of communication between the patient and the person involved in providing health education. Effective communication – using the skills of active listening, open questioning and picking up verbal and non-verbal cues – is essential. In addition, there is evidence that patients' recall of information given during a consultation improves significantly if some simple rules are followed. Thus, when providing health education:

- use short words and short sentences
- organise the information into clear categories
- give instructions and advice *early* in the interview
- stress the *importance* of the advice and the instructions you give
- *repeat* the advice during the course of the interview
- give *specific* advice.

Besides using good communication skills, when giving information it is essential to ensure that there is an exchange of information and ideas between patient and educator. A health education interview can be divided into four phases:

1 Elicit the person's health beliefs.
2 *Information phase* – this is a two-way process, with the educator seeking information from the patient and at the same time providing information.
3 *Negotiating phase* – if the patient decides to make a change then an achievable and realistic target must be discussed, choices offered and action agreed. The desirability for continued support is then discussed.
4 *Promoting change* – ways of promoting change include support from family and friends, ways in which the individual can recognise the achievement with 'self-rewards' and perhaps general changes in lifestyle.

Ideally, health education should be part of every consultation, although this is limited by the time available. A study of the process and content of consultations of varying length found that GPs were more likely to give health education advice in the longer (10-min) than in the shorter (5-min) consultation (Morrell et al 1986). Practice nurses play an important part in providing health education and might be more effective because they may have more time available and patients could feel more comfortable discussing their lifestyle with the nurse. Training in health education techniques should be provided for staff carrying out this important role.

Studies have shown that reinforcing the verbal advice with appropriate pamphlets helps the patient to retain information and make choices. Health education resources, including pamphlets and videos, are usually available from local health promotion units.

> **L** What do you think is the role of the GP in addressing non-medical or social causes of ill health, such as poverty, malnutrition or health inequality?

The ethics of prevention and health promotion

A detailed discussion of the ethics of prevention is beyond the scope of this chapter (for further reading in this area see Downie & Calman 1987). Remember that in prevention, just as in the treatment of disease, we have a duty to:

- ensure that the benefit of any procedure outweighs any possible harm to the patient
- respect the patient's autonomy
- distribute our resources fairly.

Further discussion of these principles can be found in Chapters 13–15. It is particularly important to follow these basic ethical principles in preventive activities when it is usually the doctor, rather than the patient, who initiates the activity.

Summary

- The prevention of disease and promotion of health are core activities of GPs and primary health teams, but responsibility lies also with government and society as a whole.

- Health promotion aims to enhance positive health and to prevent ill health through the overlapping spheres of health education, prevention and health protection.

- Preventive activities can be classified as primary prevention (removing the cause of disease), secondary prevention (screening) or tertiary prevention (preventing disability from established disease).

- The key areas for prevention identified in *The Health of the Nation* are coronary heart disease and stroke, cancers, mental illness, HIV/AIDS and sexual health and accidents.

- The Governments's programme of National Service Frameworks (NSFs) (e.g. for mental health, coronary heart disease and diabetes) puts significant emphasis on prevention. There are concerns as to how primary care will cope with the increasing workload as more frameworks emerge.

- The primary healthcare team has an important role to play in the preventive care of both 'high-risk' individuals and the whole practice population.

- A screening test aims to identify a disease or its precursor in an asymptomatic individual. It is not a diagnostic test. Screening programmes should be evaluated carefully before being introduced into the practice.

- Health education aims to diminish ill health and enhance positive health by influencing people's beliefs, attitudes and behaviour. It involves more than giving information: it is helping people to take control over decisions that affect their health.

- Ethical considerations must be involved in prevention. As health professionals, we have a duty to ensure that the benefit of any procedure outweighs any possible harm to the patient, to respect the patient's autonomy and to distribute our resources fairly.

> **L** How would you apportion responsibility for health promotion between GP, patient, primary healthcare team, other professions and the State?

References

Downie RS, Calman KC 1987 Healthy respect. Ethics in health care. Faber & Faber, London

Downie RS, Fyfe C, Tannahill A 1990 Health promotion: models and values. Oxford University Press, Oxford

Holland WW, Stewart S 1990 Screening in health care. Nuffield Provincial Hospitals Trust, Oxford

Last JM 1963 The iceberg. Completing the clinical picture in general practice. Lancet 2:28–31

Morrell DC, Evans ME, Morris RW, Roland MO 1986 The 'five minute' consultation: effect of time constraint on clinical content and patient satisfaction. British Medical Journal 292:870–873

Secretary of State for Health 1992 The health of the nation: a strategy for health in England. HMSO, London

Secretary of State for Health 1998 A first class service: quality in the new NHS. HMSO, London. Online. Available: http://www.doh.gov.uk/newnhs/quality.htm

Secretary of State for Health 1997 The New NHS, modern, dependable. HMSO, London. Online. Available: http://www.archive.official-documents.co.uk/ document/doh/newnhs/contents.htm

Secretary of State for Health 2000 The NHS plan. A plan for investment, a plan for reform. HMSO, London. Online. Available: http://www.nhs.uk/nationalplan/

South East London Screening Study Group 1977 A controlled trial of multi-phasic screening in middle-age: results of the South East London Screening Study. International Journal of Epidemiology 6: 357–363

Section 3

Quality in practice

8 What is clinical governance?

Jeannette Naish

Quality in practice

There is wide variation in the quality of practice from what has been called 'leading' edge to 'trailing' edge. The social, demographic and geographic characteristics of the patient population, the organisation and resources for service delivery and the commitment and clinical interest of primary healthcare professionals are some of the factors that could affect the quality of care that patients receive. The World Health Organization (WHO) considers quality of care under four broad headings:

1 professional performance
2 resource usage
3 risk management
4 patient satisfaction.

Improving the quality of clinical care depends on the commitment of individual clinicians and clinical teams to deliver patient care of the highest quality. Measuring quality of care is complex, so that the four aspects of care set out by the WHO are useful parameters for consideration.

Professional performance refers to technical quality, where clinical and communication skills are closely inter-related, supported by a caring approach and evidence-based practice.

Resource usage can be thought of as efficiency and effectiveness, where efficient organisation for service delivery complements the choice of effective interventions.

Risk management concerns minimising risk of injury or illness associated with service delivery. This issue should be considered not only in relation to patient care, but also for the health and safety of healthcare workers.

Patient satisfaction with services provided is perhaps the most important outcome measure for high-quality care, but includes other outcomes such as effective and efficient interventions of any kind, health gains and well-being. Within the context of British general practice, continuity of care would be an important issue to consider as a thread running through all four components.

Chapters 8–12 discuss the framework in which quality in practice is considered. The components for supporting and measuring good practice need to be thought of within a context of rapid scientific and technological advancement where knowledge of the basic medical sciences and lifelong learning would enable the practitioner to keep abreast of future developments.

What is clinical governance?

Clinical governance is defined as 'A framework through which NHS organisations are accountable for continuously improving the quality of their services and safeguarding high standards of care by creating an environment in which excellence in clinical care will flourish' (NHS Executive 1999). Recent innovations for the NHS state that the key policy principles for modernisation of the health service and improving quality will be driven by standards of care set at the national level. Structures for delivering services of the highest quality and systems for quality assurance have to be set in place. This will be a dynamic process, which has to be clearly demonstrated by all organisations responsible for delivering healthcare services.

Summary of quality framework

■ Arrangements for setting clear national quality standards, through National Service Frameworks (NSFs) and the National Institute for Clinical Excellence (NICE).

■ Mechanisms for ensuring local delivery of high-quality clinical services through clinical governance reinforced by a new statutory duty of quality and supported by programmes of lifelong learning and local delivery of professional self-regulation.

■ Effective systems for monitoring delivery of quality standards, in the form of a new statutory Commission for Health Improvement and an NHS Performance Assessment Framework, together with the first national survey of patient and user experience.

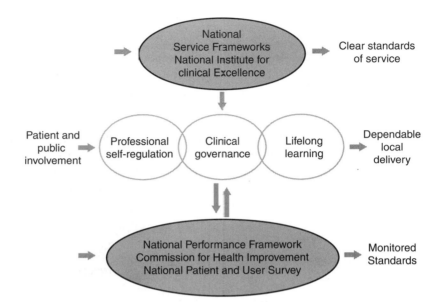

Figure 8.1
What the quality framework means for patients (NHS Executive 1999).

The concept of accountability and continuously improving and sustaining high standards of care is crucial to this strategy for improving the quality of patient care (Fig. 8.1). Implementation of the agenda would require the successful development and delivery of clinical governance. This might seem abstract and somewhat remote from the registrar learning the craft of general practice. But it is to be hoped that this 'environment in which excellence in clinical care will flourish' will become the norm in the professional lives of present and future general practitioners.

> **L** In this, as in some other matters, the administrative and regulatory frameworks are not the same in the four countries comprising the United Kingdom. Regardless of where you happen to practise, you should be aware of the main regional variations.

Clinical governance and primary care

General practice, as an NHS organisation, will be accountable to the public, with an opportunity to create an environment of excellence. Primary Care Groups and Trusts, individual general practitioners, practices and primary care teams, are all accountable. It has been stated that clinical governance 'will mean the creation of a systematic set of mechanisms that will support staff and develop all health organisations to deliver a new approach to quality'. This includes general practice. Guidance for Primary Care Groups published by the NHS Executive in June 1999 described the main components of clinical governance as:

- clear lines of responsibility and accountability for the overall quality of clinical care
- a comprehensive programme of quality improvement systems (including clinical audit, supporting and applying evidence-based practice,

implementing clinical standards and guidelines, workforce planning and development)
- education and training plans
- clear policies aimed at managing risk
- integrated procedures for all professional groups to identify and remedy poor performance.

Clinical governance is therefore about a process to establish the systems for monitoring the delivery of care to assure quality and to demonstrate that the systems for delivering high-quality care are in place. Whereas good practice and success will be celebrated, failure to achieve acceptable standards of care will need to be remedied. Responsibility for delivering a high-quality service lies at all levels of service delivery, with the:

- individual (doctor, nurse, receptionist, manager)
- primary care team
- Primary Care Group/Trust
- Health Authority
- NHS Executive.

The general practice perspective

The traditional independent contractor status of general practitioners implies that each practice is an organisation for delivering and providing healthcare services. Like all other healthcare organisations in the NHS, clinical governance is about fostering a culture of excellence in which the best care can be delivered to patients. The requirement to become more accountable and to perform regular clinical audit was contained in the 1990 Contract for General Practitioners in the NHS. Implicit in accountability is the critical appraisal of performance and the threat of sanctions for failing to achieve set standards, where poor performance requires remedial action. How then, could performance be measured?

Performance indicators

Indicators for measuring technical performance have been proposed for general practice. Altogether, over 200 separate indicators have been identified at some time as potentially valid markers of the quality of general practice care, covering both organisational and clinical areas (see Table 8.1 for examples). These cover access and organisational performance reflecting effectiveness of resource use, a limited range of chronic diseases, prescribing and gate keeping. These indicators can only partially measure the quality of general practice services, being markers, or proxies, for indirectly measuring the efficiency of service delivery. The patient–doctor relationship, individual diagnostic and therapeutic skills, consultation skills, commitment to the community and professional integrity are not so easy to measure, needing more direct observation and over time. Some performance indicators are designed to

Table 8.1
Examples of performance indicators for general practice

Area to be measured	Performance indicator
Access	Waiting time for routine appointment
Organisational performance	Numbers and categories of employed staff
Target payments	Cervical cytology uptake rate Immunisation uptake rate (child and adult)
Health promotion	Range of clinics such as asthma, diabetes, child health
Prescribing	Percentage of items prescribed generically Ratio of inhaled steroids and cromoglycates to bronchodilators
Hospital referral rates (gate keeping)	Hospital admissions, outpatient referrals

reward higher levels of performance and others are minimum standards with which all practices must comply.

> **L** Give examples of some outcome measures that you consider are valid and reliable performance indicators, and also of some in current use that are less sound. What alternatives could you suggest, and what might be the problems in adopting them?

There are, however, financial incentives for meeting performance targets; for example, in prescribing incentive schemes, cervical cytology screening uptake, child immunisation uptake and influenza vaccination among others. Other performance indicators, at a Health District or Primary Care Trust level, are selected as measures of the size of a health problem. For example, the prescribing indicators, asthma, diabetes or epilepsy admission rates might be used as proxies for the burden of health care, or health outcomes, and might partially reflect the quality of clinical practice. These indicators or targets are set nationally, and are all affected to some degree by factors outside the control of the individual clinician or the health service. Socioeconomic conditions of the population, the supply or availability of hospital beds and admission policies could all have an influence on whether performance targets are met. High levels of poverty and population mobility in some areas affect the attainment of performance targets to the extent that practices have great difficulty in achieving the higher targets, thus making the performance indicator a disincentive. Furthermore, these effects vary across geographic areas. Therefore, indicators of professional performance, measuring technical quality within the control of the clinician, should not be confused with health outcomes (Giuffrida et al 1999).

Some aspects of primary care performance indicators reflect the need to measure resource usage. For example, the time patients have to wait for an appointment might reflect the availability of the doctor but is also an outcome measure for the organisation and resource use by the practice. Setting a standard for waiting time for routine appointments might be a target at which a practice could aim when reviewing and planning resource use. Similarly, the ability to attain targets for cervical screening coverage or child immunisation needs an efficient organisational infrastructure.

The leadership potential of employees

The implementation of clinical governance within a practice requires the support of an organisation and infrastructure, with effective and efficient operational systems enabling the delivery of high-quality patient care. The whole practice will contribute towards delivering a high-quality service in partnership with the wider primary care team. There will be many individuals in the practice team, particularly practice nurses and managers, who will be more than able to direct the activities of the doctors. Their clinical and management skills often contribute to a better range and quality of patient services, and incidentally an increase in practice profit. They are sometimes not valued to the degree that they should be and practices can sometimes find themselves with a hierarchical system where the employer is in command. A change in the practice management culture might be necessary to enable true partnership working; the evaluation of Personal Medical Services (PMS) pilot schemes may give some answers. It is also important that systems for monitoring the delivery of care try to ensure that quality extends beyond the practice.

A multiagency perspective

The stated focus of clinical governance is the delivery of high-quality care to service users and carers. At the service level in primary care, as elsewhere, clinical teams will have shared responsibility for delivering effective and efficient, high-quality patient care. There is also the imperative that teams should analyse and assess the quality of their services to seek ways for improvement, in other words, audit. These activities will need to be multidisciplinary and multiagency; particularly in the continuing care of people with chronic or disabling conditions. Specific examples spanning the primary and secondary care interface are diabetes mellitus, asthma and epilepsy. Care groups such as older people and people with mental illness are further examples where multisectoral and multiprofessional care of high quality need to be delivered seamlessly for patients. Community and social care professionals have essential roles to play, yet accountability for the quality of care links back to the service-providing agencies.

It could be that in this changing climate of clinical effectiveness and the pursuit of clinical excellence, 'shared governance' will become the order of the day. Collective responsibility and accountability will have to be shared by all members of the team, and providers, including administrative members.

Good communication will always be the cornerstone of true partnership and team working. The converse – miscommunication – frequently underlies dysfunctional teams and service failures. The general requirements for achieving successful shared governance have much in common with the components for true teamwork:

- sharing a common understanding of the aims and objectives of the service to be delivered
- sharing a common understanding of how a team should work
- sharing a common understanding of the professional roles and responsibilities
- sharing an understanding of professional cultures
- sharing a mutual respect and trust for the professional judgement of another member of the team
- sharing a culture of collaboration, cooperation and coordination
- valuing the strengths and weaknesses of individuals
- sharing an understanding of the meaning of clear lines of responsibility and communication within the team
- sharing an understanding of the requirements of clinical governance.

L Why do some primary care teams seem to function more harmoniously and effectively than others? What are the signs that a team is performing suboptimally? What strategies can you suggest to improve matters? (Suggested reading: Belbin 1981).

Sharing standards and audit

The processes for achieving shared governance need to address the issues of how clinical teams and organisations could assess the quality of services to patients and carers, identify areas for improvement, promote collaborative innovations, evaluate the effectiveness of resource use and monitor the quality of care. For example, practice clinical meetings to develop practice policy on how to manage minor, self-limiting illnesses could include practice nurses, managers, receptionists, health visitors, district nurses and the local pharmacist. These could become regular opportunities for shared learning, reviewing evidence and audit. Try it and see.

A quality improvement process

From the starting point of setting in place the systems for delivering a high-quality service and for monitoring quality of care in a practice team, comparing and sharing information about practice performance with *other* practice teams would allow practices to reflect upon their performance relative to their peers. In a mutually supportive and facilitative culture, this should enable continuing improvement in standards of clinical care for a wide spectrum of clinical conditions. Practices willing to implement change to improve the outcomes from comparative audit information would be really closing the audit loop (see Chapter 10). Of course, resources for information technology, data collection and training will be necessary. The data on practice computer systems might not be of a high quality initially, so that audit data showing poor performance might not reflect the quality of clinical care but instead the quality of data recording and collection! A culture change might be needed, where the use of data to measure performance becomes part of clinical routine, no longer separate from its use for claiming target payments or staff reimbursements.

> **L** What demands does clinical governance make upon information technology and data handling procedures? What improvements in these areas might be necessary for clinical governance to have the best impact on patient care?

The whole process of quality improvement must be about getting good and better. Sharing learning and information to disseminate good practice and innovations will be key features to raising standards. Transparency in agreed clinical risk-reduction systems where adverse events, whether serious or trivial, would be detected and discussed openly would be a visible way to assure quality (see Chapter 11).

Clinical governance: the agenda for learning

The central theme for clinical governance is raising the standards of patient care. Associated with this are many strands, of which extending the health professional's responsibilities from the individual to collective team responsibility is pivotal. All health professionals will need to learn how to work effectively in teams, to assess the performance of the team and to improve the quality of services to patients within a culture of excellence. The learning agenda therefore needs to cover the knowledge, skills and attitudes required for implementing the principal components for the successful achievement of shared governance.

Overall standards for the quality of patient-centred care will be determined nationally by the NSFs and NICE, to raise standards of services and reduce unacceptable inequalities in health and social care. These will be delivered through clinical governance, underpinned by lifelong learning and professional regulation, and monitored by the Commission for Health Improvement (CHI), a Performance Assessment Framework and a programme of patient and user surveys. However, there could be local standards agreed within the community of GPs and developed in partnership with the secondary sector that complement the NSF, and ensure that implementation has the support of colleagues in the hospital sector.

Educational components for clinical governance

The extension of a clinician's individual responsibility for the patient to collective, or corporate, responsibility for a service to patients goes beyond the concepts embodied in the Hippocratic Oath. This extension will require a change in culture and all the learning that goes with it. Equally, there will be an extension of corporate accountability in management to clinical accountability in medical practice. This extension of responsibility has been acknowledged and recognised by the General Medical Council. The challenges presented by the move from traditional forms of continuing medical education to continuing professional development for whole clinical teams are considerable. Multiprofessional learning and performance monitoring will require new skills and resources. Audit and assessment will be key components in this procedure. One objective for audit will be the detection of adverse events. The skill to assess the nature of the problem, to perform a critical analysis of patient complaints or adverse events, and to learn from mistakes is essential. How to deal with poor performance by clinicians becomes part of the role of clinical governance leaders, needing further educational resources for remedial action and managerial resources to facilitate the process. The whole process must lead to the establishment of a culture of lifelong professional learning (see Chapter 12).

The agenda for learning through clinical governance can be summarised to cover:

- communication skills for true team work (including work at the primary/secondary and the health/social care interface)
- critical appraisal of performance and evidence, to enable the understanding and implementation of good clinical practice and to learn from failures in standards of care
- audit to monitor standards of clinical care and to detect adverse events
- clinical risk management.

Suggested areas for reflection

It has been suggested that Primary Care Groups (and Trusts) should support best practice through incentive schemes with the aim of developing high-quality primary and community health services (Hasler et al 1991). Registrars would benefit from focusing on the 10 points of clinical governance for primary care contained in *The New NHS* (NHS Executive 1998). These could be tutorial topics, subjects for discussion and reflection during the half-day release scheme, or areas for further reading or audit:

1 Quality improvement processes (e.g. clinical audit) are in place and integrated with the quality programme for the organisation as a whole:
   - What does 'integrated' mean?
   - What are the 'processes' and are they in place?
   - How does it work in your practice?
   - How do other practices do it?
2 Leadership skills are developed at clinical team level:
   - Observation during a primary care team meeting: use the list of components for true teamwork to evaluate the dynamics within the team.

- Is it really working as a team?
- What is the role of the GP, and how is it being performed?
- Does it enable the development of leadership skills by all members of the team?

3 Evidence-based practice is in day-to-day use with the infrastructure to support it:

- This is a rich area for audit.
- As a starting point, focus on the infrastructure. See what there is in your practice, talk about this with your colleagues on the half-day release scheme and see if you can come up with an 'ideal' situation or a standard that could be used to audit your own practice.

4 Good practice, ideas and innovations (which have been evaluated) are disseminated systematically within and outside organisations:

- How are good practice, ideas and innovations evaluated?
- What are the overall objectives for the personal and practice development programmes in your practice? How are they operationalised? Are the objectives really being met?
- What are the overall objectives for the programme at the local Academic Centre? Obtain a copy of the programme and think about it critically and see if it fulfils this requirement.

5 Clinical risk reduction programmes are in place. The subject of risk management is discussed in Chapter 11 but it might be interesting to start by:

- Talking to the practice manager about the health and safety procedures in the practice, discuss and compare differences between practices with your vocational training scheme (VTS) colleagues.
- Discussing operational systems for appointments and home visits with your practice manager. Are there written protocols in place? Talk to your VTS colleagues. Are there 'gaps' in the systems so that mistakes might occur? Is there duplication in the systems so that there is inefficient use of resources?

6 Adverse events are detected, openly investigated and learning applied. This is again part of risk management. There should, however, be a patient complaints procedure in place. Find out about this from your practice manager:

- Are patient complaints audited?
- Are complaints analysed using a risk management protocol?

7 Problems of poor clinical performance are recognised at an early stage and dealt with both to prevent harm to patients and to improve the practitioner's development. This is in some ways related to patient complaints. However, poor clinical performance by an individual GP in a large group practice can be masked or diluted. It really behoves the other partners to address the issue of poor or worse, risky clinical performance by a partner. This could become more complicated for smaller practices. Remember Harold Shipman:

- Do GPs own up to clinical mistakes? How are these handled?

8 Lessons for clinical practice are systematically learned from the input of patients. Positive feedback from patients is probably the most useful form of reinforcement for good practice. Negative feedback is never easy to handle, particularly if this provokes defensiveness or conflict. However, complaints could be constructive if handled sensitively and critically. A systematic analysis of the complaint would yield many lessons:

■ What are the gaps in lines of communication between a patient arriving at the reception desk demanding to see a doctor when there is no doctor on the premises?

9 All professional development programmes reflect the principles of clinical governance. This is similar to point 4. Critically appraise professional development programmes to see if they truly facilitate 'a framework through which NHS organisations (in this case general practice and GPs) are accountable for continuously improving the quality of their services and safeguarding high standards of care by creating an environment in which excellence in clinical care will flourish'.

10 The quality of data gathered to monitor clinical care is itself of a high standard. Most operational systems for collecting data in general practice originated as administrative systems for claiming fees and allowances. These were later adapted for collecting clinical data:

■ What systems are in place in your practice for managing the payroll, claims, appointments?

■ How do administrative systems relate to basic patient registration information?

■ What clinical functions are computerised?

■ How would you construct a disease register (e.g. asthma) from the available data in your practice?

■ How good is the clinical data in your practice?

L Are you clear in your mind what the phrase 'clinical governance' means? (Is *anybody*? And if not, why not?) What factors do you think have led to the concept assuming prominence in the last few years? Why do you think some GPs are critical or sceptical about it?

Summary

■ Clinical governance provides a framework through which NHS organisations strive for continuous improvement in the quality of their services and standards of care.

■ The main components of clinical governance are: clear lines of responsibility and accountability, a programme of quality improvement, education and training plans, policies to manage risk and procedures to identify and remedy poor performance.

■ For general practice, clinical governance means that all members of the practice team will undergo critical appraisal of their performance.

■ In the general practice setting, performance can be measured through performance indicators, which cover both organisational and clinical areas.

■ Computer systems will be valuable tools in the improvement of quality in the general practice setting.

References

Belbin RM 1981 Management teams: why they suceed or fail. Heinemann, Oxford

Giuffrida A, Gravelle H, Roland M 1999 Measuring quality of care with routine data: avoiding confusion between performance indicators and health outcomes. British Medical Journal 319: 94–98

Hasler J, Bryceland C, Hobden-Clarke L, Moreton P 1991 Handbook of practice management. Churchill Livingstone, Edinburgh

NHS Executive 1998 The new NHS: a national framework for assessing performance. Department of Health, London

NHS Executive 1999 Clinical governance: quality in the new NHS. Health Service Circular. Department of Health, London

9 Evidence-based practice and clinical guidelines

Jeannette Naish

'Evidence-based' practice, medicine, health care, policy, guidelines and thinking are now familiar ideas. The basic idea that what we do as healthcare providers should be based, as far as possible, on sound evidence is neither new nor controversial. However, many decisions made by rushed GPs in busy surgeries are still based on 'experience', 'expert opinion', 'rules of thumb' and 'anecdotes'. This is to a large extent inevitable because instant 'scientific' evidence in primary care is not always available or practical to follow. Many of the problems we deal with are complex, multifactorial and largely unresearched. Medical decisions must take into account the individual patient and her or his personal circumstances, social and psychological background and, to some extent, public policy, but these issues are not easily taken into account in clinical trials (Starfield 2001).

It is, however, important to know that a body of evidence exists to support many of our decisions, whether for individual patients or at a policy level. It is also essential for the modern GP to be skilled in efficient methods of accessing and appraising the evidence. In an ideal world, when we are considering a clinical decision at either individual or practice level the important questions to ask are:

- Is there evidence to help me decide what is the best action to recommend?
- Where is the evidence and how do I access it?
- What does the evidence show?
- Is the quality of the evidence good enough for me to take into account?
- Does the evidence apply to my particular patient or population?

What is evidence-based medicine?

Evidence-based medicine, according to one of its major proponents, David Sackett (1996) 'is about integrating individual clinical expertise and the best external evidence'. It would be worthwhile taking some time to reflect upon the meaning and application of this statement. Clinical expertise is about the skill to make the best clinical decision for the patient and to help the patient to make choices about his or her treatment. There are many components in the process of making clinical decisions. Some have good external scientific evidence in support, others have little or none.

Clinical expertise and best external evidence

Clinical expertise is built on basic clinical skills, then derived from experience and expressed as judgement when making clinical decisions. But experience is acquired not only from what one learns through practising these skills, but also through anecdotal evidence and a sharing of 'expert' opinion, all of which are hard to quantify or measure. The last two components of learning are often derided, but make up a large part of a wider view of the practice of medicine as an art supported by science.

The best available external evidence is clinically relevant research derived from patient-centred research and basic medical sciences. This covers the accuracy of diagnostic and screening tests, identifying risk factors and prognostic markers, and evaluating the efficacy and safety of therapeutic, preventive and rehabilitative interventions. The 'evidence' in support of evidence-based medicine is mostly quantitative, in the form of randomised controlled trials, emphasising the quantifiable and measurable aspects of medical practice. In a real-life situation there will be areas of clinical uncertainty. The less easily measured factors that influence clinical decisions, such as the psychological and social condition of the patient, might in fact be more important and only to be ignored at the doctor's peril. So many forms of evidence, including anecdotal and qualitative evidence, support clinical decisions. For example, a large-enough series of anecdotes about a single condition would make a descriptive series of case reports giving insights into the natural history of the condition. The discipline of evidence-based medicine is important for some aspects of clinical decision making, some of which relate more to an overall strategy for managing a population of patients, for example people with diabetes, and some that will relate to economic choices of cost-effective strategies. It would be worthwhile to reflect upon these aspects, and their relevance to the preferences of the patient sitting in front of you.

Diagnosis and treatment

The following case illustrations might help your understanding of how you make clinical decisions and where 'best external evidence' might come in.

Case illustrations

How can you tell if the hot 3-year-old who has been coughing and spluttering for the last 12 h has the beginnings of a pneumococcal infection? How confident can you be that 'It's only a virus'? What evidence is there to support your diagnostic decision? Is there a way for improving the clinical diagnosis of pneumococcal infection?

The likelihood is that the majority of GPs will not take nasal aspirates or serology but will wait and see if the child gets better or sicker without making the diagnosis. Equally likely is that the child will be prescribed an antibiotic if he or she is brought back 24 h later. Why do GPs prescribe antibiotics for what is potentially a viral infection and for which there is no evidence to suggest that antibiotics are effective?

You have been asked by your trainer to work out some options for diabetic retinopathy screening for the population of type II diabetics that the practice looks after.

What kinds of evidence would you need before you can make a start? Would you go for evidence about the accuracy and effectiveness of different screening tests first or would you think about your patient population first? What is the prevalence of type II diabetes in the practice? What are the social and economic conditions and educational attainment of your patients? What is the geographic location of the practice (you might be next door to a specialised ophthalmology unit or the nearest optician could be 15 miles away)? What services are available for patients with diabetic retinopathy? You will see that some of the evidence you need for this type of decision has to be based on your experience of local conditions, and is specific to local conditions. Evidence from trials can give you the information on which the best screening test is in terms of identifying early retinopathy accurately but there might be practical and economic constraints on using this test for screening the population of type II diabetics, so that the chosen test might have to be second best. Evidence from trials can also give information about how screening could reduce the risk of blindness in type II diabetics. Convincing your patients that regular screening is worthwhile can be difficult if their eyesight appears perfectly normal to them and if attending for screening means that they have to make an appointment, take time off work and travel 15 miles to the nearest centre.

Is the evidence good enough? Critical appraisal of evidence

Having reflected upon the place of evidence in medicine, we now need to consider whether a given piece of evidence is good enough to support a clinical decision: we must critically appraise the evidence. This is not about picking faults in a piece of published research but about the application of certain rules of evidence to clinical, epidemiological and other published data to determine their validity and applicability. A good start to understanding the approach of clinical epidemiology and reflecting upon the scientific principles underlying the art of clinical medicine, is to read *Clinical epidemiology – a basic science for clinical medicine* (Sackett et al 1991).

Try to practise your basic critical appraisal skills by applying them throughout the training year. As well as thinking about how you read journal articles, this approach should be applied to evidence supporting clinical guidelines and treatment protocols, evidence supporting the pharmaceutical industry's recommendation to prescribe one particular medicine in preference to another, evidence for public health policies and service-commissioning strategies. The practice of critically appraising evidence put before us should be a lifelong activity. As doctors, we are constantly doing this when trying to make medical sense of the evidence that patients bring to us. However, most of us are not used to reading the medical literature critically, not least because there is so much of it.

Detailed advice on how to appraise all kinds of published research can be found in a number of books (see Further reading). Greenhalgh gives useful guidance in *How to Read a Paper* (Greenhalgh 1997). You might also consider taking one of a number of short courses on critical appraisal available around the country.

When appraising any research paper there are essentially four central questions that you should apply:

1 What is this research about? (i.e. is the research question clear?)
2 Was a valid method used to answer the research question?
3 What are the results?
4 How do the results apply to *your* patients?

What is this research about?

Any research must start with a clearly stated research question. Sometimes this is obvious from the title of the paper. If not, look for aims or objectives in the abstract section. If there is no abstract, check towards the end of the introduction. If you are still not clear what the research question is then there might well be a problem with the paper. If the question is clear but of no relevance to you, then you might choose not to read the paper.

Was a valid method used to answer the research question?

There are basically two main types of research:

1 quantitative studies, which are numerical and based on epidemiological methods
2 qualitative studies, which collect information in non-numerical forms (e.g. interview data or analysis of written text).

Quantitative studies

Quantitative studies can be descriptive or experimental. Both are important although the randomised controlled trial has often been cited as the 'gold standard' in experimental study design. There are different types of quantitative study:

1 *Cross-sectional studies* – are descriptive of what is happening at a point in time. The kind of question this method is good at answering would be something like 'what is the proportion of patients with type II diabetes who have coronary heart disease?' Cross-sectional studies provide a 'snapshot'; this could take the form of a questionnaire administered to a large group of patients or analysis of information held on computer or in patient notes at one particular time.

2 *Retrospective studies* – look backwards in time to find out what happened to people with a particular condition. For example, the question 'Is there a relationship between smoking and coronary heart disease in patients with type II diabetes?' requires a retrospective, descriptive, case-controlled study. Type II diabetics with heart disease (cases) and without heart disease (controls) would be identified. Their case histories over many years would be examined to see if they smoked or not.

3 *Prospective or longitudinal studies* – look forwards in time to find out how diseases behave, and what might be associated with a more or less rapid progression. An example would be 'Is microalbuminuria a risk factor for retinopathy and nephropathy in type II diabetics?'. This would involve identifying a group, or *cohort*, of patients with type II diabetes, finding out who had microalbuminuria and who had not, then following them up over a long period of time to see who develops retinopathy or nephropathy. These are also descriptive or observational studies.

4 *Controlled trials* – study the effects of interventions of some kind and are experimental in the sense that they try to demonstrate the effectiveness or otherwise of a 'new' treatment. Classically, in a randomised controlled trial (RCT), patients are allocated randomly to receive the experimental treatment, no treatment (placebo) or the 'old' treatment. The effects are measured and compared to see if there are differences in the different groups, if the differences are statistically significant, and if the differences are clinically important.

Qualitative studies

Qualitative studies explore issues in more depth, often by semistructured face-to-face interviews with individuals or groups of subjects. Conducted rigorously and using the appropriate methodology, qualitative studies can provide useful insights into very important questions, for example 'What are the barriers to implementing national guidelines to local practice?' and 'What do patients think about self-management protocols for asthma?' There is a body of research devoted to how people perceive their state of health and how they deal with illness (see Chapter 5), providing evidence for how we might best 'promote' health. Public health strategies should be based on these types of evidence rather than relying solely on randomised controlled trials.

Choosing the right method

The choice of research method will depend on the type of question being asked, the previous knowledge available in the subject area and the approach of the researchers. Different approaches to critical appraisal are required for each different kind of study; these are all described in *How to Read a Paper*. The following are examples of the kinds of question that require consideration for a study on the effectiveness of an intervention:

1 *The research question* – was the research question clearly formulated and was the study design appropriate for the research question posed? As mentioned previously, a randomised controlled trial is the gold standard for experimental studies such as drug trials, but sometimes another design might be used for pragmatic reasons. The reader has to make a judgement about whether this is reasonable and acceptable.

2 *The study sample* – was every effort made to minimise bias? Was the assignment of patients to treatment groups randomised? Was the sample big enough to detect a significant difference between the groups (power calculation)?

3 *The outcomes* – were these clearly described? Were they sensible? Were they measurable?

4 *Were all the patients who entered the trail properly accounted for and attributed at its conclusion?* Was the treatment allocation to study and control groups carefully concealed? Was follow-up complete? Were patients analysed in the groups to which they were randomised (analysis by intention to treat)?

5 *Were patients, health workers and study personnel 'blind' to treatment?* This is relatively straightforward if the intervention was about something like a tablet. However, in some interventions, such as surgical intervention, the surgeon and the patient cannot be 'blind' to the intervention. In this case, the observer who looks at the outcomes could be blind.

6 *Were the groups similar at the start of the trial?* This also relates to the effectiveness of randomisation, which should give two groups – the cases and the controls – with almost identical characteristics in terms of age, sex, disease severity and lifestyle (e.g. smoking, alcohol intake) that could affect health risk. These details will be found in most published papers.

7 *Apart from the experimental intervention, were the two groups treated equally?* This may seem obvious but in some drug trials the medicines that patients obtain over-the-counter could have an influence on the outcomes.

What are the results?

1 *Was a difference found between the study group and the control group?* Were the appropriate statistical tests employed and, if a difference was found, could it have arisen by chance?

2 *How precise were the results?* This relates to having to work with samples of the population rather than the whole population (of diabetics, people with heart disease, etc.). Different samples, of different sizes, can give quite different results. To overcome this problem there is a statistical manoeuvre to calculate the possible range of results (a confidence interval). The interpretation is 'that given the sample you have, the true answer lies within this range'. A wide confidence interval (CI) implies a relatively imprecise result.

3 *How large is the difference in clinical outcomes?* In other words, is the difference in outcome good enough for you to choose the new treatment? This is often measured as the number of events per 100 treated (or untreated) patients, or the number of patients you need to treat to prevent an event (number needed to treat). The 'number needed to treat' is sometimes used as a proxy measure of the clinical significance of the intervention.

How do the results apply to your patients?

This is where the reader exercises judgement, based on experience of his or her own patients.

1 *Were the patients in the study similar to my own?* They do not have to be exactly the same, but are the differences sufficient to make you think that the new treatment will not work for your patients?

2 *Were all the clinically important outcomes considered?* Not all outcomes can be considered, as some are hard to measure. Often, death is used as a measurable and unambiguous outcome but there could be other outcomes somewhere between death and no difference in patient condition that are difficult or impossible to measure but that might be important to your patients.

3 *Are the likely benefits worth the potential harms and costs?* This question applies to populations as much as to individual patients. The overall costs of a treatment programme might outweigh the benefits. An example is the decision not to use lipid-lowering drugs in the primary prevention of coronary heart disease.

It might be worth joining a short course in research methods and statistics to help 'demystify' these important concepts.

L MRCGP candidates are often anxious about the level of statistical knowledge they are expected to have. Consult the Examination Regulations for guidance and examples. A working grasp of the following is recommended:

- Specificity and sensitivity; absolute risk (AR), AR increase and AR reduction; relative risk increase and reduction; hazard ratio;

> positive and negative predictive value; number needed to
> treat/harm; odds; odds ratio.
> - Basic statistical concepts including representativeness of the
>   sample; inclusion and exclusion criteria; bias; prevalence;
>   confidence intervals; probability and correlation coefficients.
> - Principles of research design; qualitative and quantitative
>   research; prospective and retrospective studies; limitations and
>   strengths of research methodologies (e.g. case control, cohort,
>   pilot studies, questionnaire design, randomised controlled trials).
> - Methodology of systematic reviews and meta-analysis.
> - Issues relating to interpretation of results including validity,
>   reliability and generalisability.

Where is the evidence?

The sheer volume of published material that might be of direct import-ance to clinical medicine makes it impossible to try to read everything. It is, however, important to foster a habit of regularly reading those journals that are most likely to publish articles that are relevant to you to keep up-to-date in areas of medicine that are relevant and of interest. For GPs this is a daunting task because every clinical development is poten-tially relevant.

In general, the *British Medical Journal* and the *British Journal of General Practice* are highly relevant to general practice matters and 'must reads' for the MRCGP examination. *Family Practice* is a quarterly inter-national journal with interesting articles broadly relevant to primary care.

Centres for systematically reviewing the evidence to support best practice have been established in all disciplines of medicine, notably, the Cochrane Collaboration and the Centre for Reviews and Dissemin-ation at the University of York. These are important sources of informa-tion on evidence-based medicine. The York Centre has its own website (http://www.york.ac.uk). The National Electronic Library for Health con-tains information about recent developments and information about useful sources of information (http://www.nelh.nhs.uk/). Evidence-based journals have also grown in number, some accessible electronically via the internet, to help you to identify the information you need to give the best and most effective management for your patients; *Evidence-based Medicine,* published by the BMJ Publishing Group, is one such.

There are also electronic databases that you can search for published evidence of interest to whatever clinical decision that you have to make. Listed below are some of the important ones:

- Medline is perhaps the most familiar (also PubMed).
- The National Research Register is a register of ongoing and recently completed research projects funded by the National Health Service.
- Best Evidence is a full-text database containing the following journals:
  - *ACP Journal Club* (1991 to date; American College of Physicians)
  - *Evidence-Based Medicine* (1995 to date).

- CHAIN (Contact, Help, Advice and Information Network) is a multi-professional network for people interested in, and involved in, evidence-based health care in the NHS.
- The Cochrane Library is a collection of three major databases:
  - the Cochrane Controlled Trials Register
  - the Cochrane Database of Systematic Reviews, which contains the full-text systematic reviews commissioned for the Cochrane Collaboration
  - DARE (Database of Abstracts of Reviews of Effectiveness), which covers quality reviews published in the medical literature.

  The Cochrane Library also includes the Health Technology Assessment database.

There are courses on how to search for literature and how to appraise and update your evidence, often as part of evidence-based medicine courses, but libraries (e.g. the British Library) will sometimes run these courses if there is enough demand. Librarians are usually extremely helpful.

Guidelines and protocols

Guidelines have, and will increasingly, become integral parts of medical practice. They are 'systematically developed statements to assist practitioner and patient decisions about appropriate health care for specific clinical circumstances' (Jackson & Feder 1998). Clinical guidelines are generally developed from evidence of effective interventions, which are then translated into guidelines through consensus. They might contain explicit and concise guidance on which diagnostic or screening procedures to follow and when, which management options to offer and when, when to refer and to whom, and other details of health care. It has to be acknowledged that the growth of the guidelines industry began with the realisation that most healthcare systems cannot meet the rising costs of increasing patient demand and expectations, the rapid proliferation of new and ever costlier technologies and an ageing population. There is also the presumption that variation in service delivery by GPs, hospital providers and geographical areas might, at least in part, be due to variation in clinical practice – that there might be inappropriate overuse or underuse of services. Patients with the same complaint might receive different treatment depending on where they live, the hospital they use and the clinician, including the GP, who is caring for them.

Clinical guidelines can be instrumental in standardising care, thereby reducing unacceptable variations in the quality of care, increasing the effectiveness and efficiency of healthcare delivery and reducing inequalities in access to services. Also through standardisation, efficiency could improve towards achieving equitable health outcomes from limited resources. For example, prescribing guidelines could reduce the cost of treatment for indigestion and guidelines for hospital referrals of skin lesions could reduce waiting times. The series of articles published in the *BMJ* on issues in the development and use of clinical guidelines is well worth reading (Feder et al 1999, Haycox et al 1999, Hurwitz 1999, Shekelle et al 1999, Woolf et al 1999).

Developing clinical guidelines

In general, guidelines have been developed based on the best available evidence on a clearly defined subject area, such as the management of diabetes or chronic back pain. The evidence is usually from systematic reviews, which pool data from equivalent studies of randomised controlled trials whenever possible. The first step would be to identify and critically appraise the evidence to see if it is good enough to inform guideline development. If, as might be expected, there are gaps in the evidence, then the next step in guideline development comes about through consensus between clinical experts. As well as external evidence, resource implications and feasibility for implementation are essential considerations when translating evidence into clinical guidelines. It is not always possible to assess the full economic implications of implementing guidelines because part of the guidance will be about better case identification, uncovering greater need and thereby increasing costs. Guidelines will need regular review in the light of new information and technology.

Clinical practice guidelines could be translated into protocols, which could be followed by all relevant members of the practice team. This is not a simple transition and might be seen as imposing a rigid requirement where variation is not tolerated, in distinction to guidelines, which are more open to voluntary use and interpretation.

The usefulness of clinical guidelines

There can be significant barriers to implementing guidelines. Some of these are attitudinal, and active education and facilitation might help doctors to understand the content of the guideline. Practice organisation and infrastructure, with poor resources, can also hinder the use of guidelines.

On the whole, rigorously constructed and user-friendly clinical practice guidelines are useful aids to clinical decision making, but it has to be said that they can only contribute to part of the decision-making process. Clinical judgement and knowledge of the patient are essential in complex clinical situations where multiple decisions may be required.

Patients could benefit from lay versions of clinical guidelines. The information could help them to make better treatment choices. It could also help them to have more realistic expectations of the outcomes of treatment.

Health service commissioners and managers, health authorities and governments also have an interest in clinical guidelines. The choice of the most cost-effective treatment might depend on the systematic reviews of treatment options contained in a guideline. For example, the NICE prescribing guidelines for interferon could inform health authority purchasing policy of interferon for multiple sclerosis patients. Clinical guidelines could also reduce unacceptable variations in standards of clinical care, and raise the overall standard of care. They might also need tools to control resource allocation through cost containment or redistribution of costs. Instruments to monitor and evaluate clinical performance could derive from clinical management protocols. The NSFs are evidence-based guidelines verging on being protocols where timeframes for meeting targets are included.

> **L** Some GPs are less than enthusiastic about the proliferation of guidelines and protocols. Why might this be?

Putting clinical guidelines into practice

To help you think about guideline implementation, the following case illustrations are suggestions for some scenarios to reflect upon. Try making up some of your own; use some broad headings to focus the processes:

- Choose a national or local guideline, or work up one of your own after reviewing external evidence. The benefit of someone else having done it already is that it saves time and effort on reviewing the evidence, but you still need to appraise the evidence in terms of 'Will it apply to my patient population?'
- Decide about whom in your practice/primary care team needs to be involved in implementing this guideline. Meet with everyone concerned to discuss the guideline and clarify roles.
- Review the target population in terms of likely workload, social and educational background, social support.
- Review the implications for the practice organisation: how will the programme for implementing *this* guideline affect practice organisation? Will it increase workload in the short or long term, and for whom? Will it decrease workload in the long term, and for whom? Will it increase efficiency in service delivery? What are the benefits for patients (don't forget health education and promotion)?

Case illustrations

> **1** The health visitors in your practice have brought you a document containing advice on diarrhoea and vomiting for children under 5 years old, for consultation. This reminds you that, when you were doing paediatrics as part of your vocational training scheme, you saw a lot of children in the Accident and Emergency Department in the early stages of gastroenteritis when oral rehydration and control of fever by the parents were the appropriate management strategy. You think that it would make sense if the health-visiting advice were built on to develop a clinical guideline for all members of the practice team that might have first contact with this problem so that management could be

standardised, with consistent advice for the parents. You also think that it might help to involve the local consultant paediatricians for some expert input and, with luck, to achieve consistency in advice given in primary and secondary care. How would you set about this?

2 Having had some experience of taking telephone calls from patients when in surgery, you note that the majority of these are for feverish children. You were at first lacking in confidence in giving advice over the telephone, so you saw all of them. But you found that what the majority of parents needed was advice about how to manage the fever and hydration, and how to observe the child for improvement or deterioration. You feel that it would be a good idea to have a guideline and a protocol for telephone advice on how to manage feverish children. How would you set about this?

3 Following the publication of the National Service Framework for diabetes, the practice feels that it needs to review the arrangements for the diabetic clinic. It is using guidelines that were developed locally 3 or 4 years ago and feels that this needs review. The practice is also unsure about how well it has covered the whole type II diabetes population and whether it meets the NSF targets in relation to clinical governance. How would you approach this problem, and how might you contribute to help the practice?

L   Knowing the evidence and being able to evaluate it is central to much of the MRCGP examination, especially the written paper and statistical sections of the MCQ. In the orals, examiners will be interested in your ability to balance rigour with healthy scepticism, and in your ability to make decisions on topics where evidence is lacking or contradictory. Common formats for questions in the written paper are 'What would be the practical implications of this paper's conclusions for your own practice? What problems might be encountered in implementing them?'

Summary
- Evidence-based medicine is the integration of clinical expertise and the best external evidence so as to make the best clinical decision for patients and to help them make choices about their care.

- Evidence-based practice means that, as far as possible, decisions are based on sound evidence.

- Although evidence is not always available in primary care, a body of evidence *does* exist to support many of the decisions made by GPs, at both the clinical and the policy level.

- Clinical guidelines are becoming integral to general practice. Their use will help to standardise care, reducing unacceptable variations in the quality of care and increasing the effectiveness and efficacy of healthcare delivery.

- It is important that guidelines are put into practice at the local level.

References

Feder G, Eccles M, Grol R et al 1999 Using clinical guidelines. British Medical Journal 318:728–730

Greenhalgh T 1997 How to read a paper. The basics of evidence-based medicine. BMJ Publishing Group, London

Haycox A, Bagust A, Walley T 1999 Clinical guidelines – the hidden costs. British Medical Journal 318:391–393

Hurwitz B 1999 Legal and political considerations of clinical practice guidelines. British Medical Journal 318:661–664

Jackson R, Feder G 1998 Guidelines for clinical guidelines. British Medical Journal 317:427–428

Sackett DL, Haynes RB, Guyatt GH, Tugwell P 1991 Clinical epidemiology – a basic science for clinical medicine. Little Brown, London

Sackett DL, Rosenberg WMC, Gray JAM et al 1996 Evidence based medicine: what it is and what it isn't. British Medical Journal 312:71–72

Shekelle PG, Woolf SH, Eccles M, Grimshaw J 1999 Developing guidelines. British Medical Journal 318:593–596

Starfield B 2001 New paradigms for quality in primary care. British Journal of General Practice 51:303–309

Woolf SH, Grol R, Hutchinson A et al 1999 Potential benefits, limitations and harms of clinical guidelines. British Medical Journal 318:527–530

Further reading

Armstrong D Grace J 2000 Research methods and audit in general practice. Oxford General Practice Series, Oxford

Bland M 2000 An introduction to medical statistics. Oxford University Press, Oxford

Coggon D 1995 Statistics in clinical practice. BMJ Publishing Group, London

Humphris D, Littlejohns P 1999 Implementing clinical guidelines: a practical guide. Radcliffe Medical Press, Oxford

Petrie A, Sabin C 2000 Medical statistics at a glance. Blackwell Science, Oxford

Sackett DL, Richardson WS, Rosenberg WMC, Haynes RB 2000 Evidence-based medicine: how to practise and teach EBM, 2nd edn. Churchill Livingstone, London

10 Clinical audit and practice-based research

Jeannette Naish

Research and audit are intimately related but not synonymous. In simple terms, research aims to answer the question 'what is right?' whereas audit aims to answer the question 'are we doing it right?'. Despite this basic difference they share many essential characteristics because in both research and audit:

- the starting point must be a well-defined question
- objectives must be clear
- measures used must be valid
- concepts to be explored must be defined operationally
- data collected must be critically analysed using accepted methods
- results and conclusions must be interpreted fairly and objectively without bias.

Both research and audit are concerned with outcomes but research seeks to determine the relationship between outcomes and structure and/or process, whereas audit assumes that outcomes are indirect proxies for appropriate structure and process, and vice versa. Other differences relate to methods, focus on individuals, populations or communities, place and time frame.

Clinical audit

An auditor is someone who listens and hears, but does not necessarily make a judgement on what is heard. In this sense, although not only through listening, clinical or medical audit is about finding out what is happening in order to make a judgement on whether this is good enough and, if not, decide what to do to make improvements. Further audit is then undertaken to find out whether improvements have taken place, what did or did not work and what more needs to be done (Fig. 10.1).

The terms 'clinical audit' and 'medical audit' are often used interchangeably but do have different technical meanings in the literature. Clinical audit covers all aspects of clinical care, including the roles of nurses, paramedical staff and in some cases administrative staff, whereas medical audit would usually address activities directly initiated by doctors.

Audit became a requirement in UK general practice when the 1990 GP Contract was introduced. Audit is seen as a powerful tool for improving the quality of patient care and providing opportunities for the education of doctors and other health professionals. The importance of audit as a fundamental part of general practice is recognised in summative assessment, which is now compulsory for all registrars in general practice. The written submission element of summative assessment is in fact commonly referred to as 'the audit' because this is the type of submission chosen by most registrars. A completed audit cycle – including the implementation of change and a second collection of data – is the favoured method in some deaneries. In this chapter we will consider the principles of audit in general practice then suggest some topics for audit that may be useful for your practice. Box 10.1 outlines 10 steps involved in conducting a practice audit.

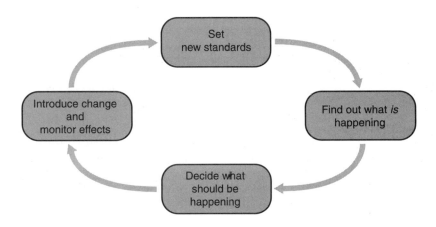

Figure 10.1
The audit cycle.

Box 10.1
10 steps in conducting a practice audit

> 1 Background – as a starting point it is helpful to clarify the problem that initiated the audit
> 2 Define the questions you wish to answer – what are the objectives of the audit?
> 3 Set criteria and standards – ideally, what should be happening?
> 4 Decide on the method to be used for finding out what is happening – what information will be collected? How will the information be collected? From whom/where? By whom?
> 5 Collect the information
> 6 Analyse the results
> 7 Compare results with the standards set
> 8 What needs to be changed?
> 9 How can we implement change?
> 10 Were the changes effective?

The principles of audit in general practice

Whether a piece of audit has been successful can be judged in terms of whether the outcome is instrumental in improving the quality of service to patients. In terms of clinical audit, the first principle has to be motivation: the enthusiasm of the auditor, the willingness of the practice, including the whole practice team, to participate in audit, and then to implement change in the light of audit findings and decisions about what changes are needed.

L What factors may limit the extent of clinical audit undertaken within a practice?

Commitment to participate in audit

To be a meaningful and professional activity, the 'right' reason for audit would be the desire, shared by all professionals, to find out about their work in relation to the quality of services and benefits to patients, and in terms of the current state-of-the-art or 'gold standard'. Other motivations no doubt exist, for example, to satisfy contractual requirements or to justify additional staff or other resources. Incentive schemes have been set up using rewards such as financial payments or provision of equipment for carrying out audits. In an ideal world such inducements to engage in audit should not be necessary, and they are not always desirable. Acknowledging that practice audit requires an organisational infrastructure and more staff time, preoccupation with material incentives misses the point that audit should benefit the patients, the doctors and whole practice team.

A more practical, but no less important, issue needing motivation is the agreement to audit a particular subject. In this respect, clinical practice guidelines, performance indicators, the National Service Frameworks, critical incidents and local needs give strong leads on topics for clinical audit, and in some cases, have set overall or national standards.

Box 10.2
Choosing a subject for audit

- Will the audit benefit patients?
- Will it benefit the practice?
- Is it important to professional development?
- Will it justify the time, effort and money invested in the project?
- Is it of sufficient interest and importance to the practice team to maintain enthusiasm?
- Does the problem have significant incidence and prevalence?
- Is there a high risk to patients if appropriate service is not delivered?
- Is there a 'gold standard' for service delivery in this case?

Choosing a subject for audit

When choosing a subject for audit, it is vital that this will demonstrate the quality of patient care being provided and have the potential for improvements. The subject should also represent a problem that is important to the practice team, and is one that they want to solve (Box 10.2).

A topic frequently encountered by the team, such as diabetes, would be more appropriate than a rare occurrence such as phaeochromocytoma. A high level of risk to patients associated with the audit topic would be of interest. For example, when there is potential patient disability associated with an absence of appropriate intervention or the presence of inappropriate intervention.

Known or suspected problems about whether the service provided in the audit topic follows current state-of-the-art advances in knowledge and technology would be of interest to the practice and a good subject for audit. Auditing the process of healthcare delivery (for a specific topic) against the state-of-the-art or 'gold standard' management also provides an excellent opportunity for shared learning with all concerned with the delivery of care. It could result in benefits for patients in the shape of more up-to-date management. It might also have implications for practice organisation and investment in better service delivery.

Types of audit topics for general practice include:

- clinical care
- prescribing
- preventive care
- practice organisation.

Areas for general practice audit have much in common with areas for research in general practice, often addressing the 'gaps' in available evidence:

- clinical
- epidemiological
- operational
- behavioural (patients and health professionals).

L Do you think the improvements in care resulting from audit are 'topic specific'? i.e. what may be the effects of auditing one aspect of care on other conditions or problems?

Box 10.3
Auditing the structure, process and outcome of diabetic care

Structure
- *Definition* – the facilities available for providing care (e.g. the building, people, equipment)
- *Objectives* – availability of urine- and blood-testing equipment; facilities for diabetic retinopathy screening; practice diabetes disease register

Process
- *Definition* – how the procedures for routine diabetic care is carried out; what is actually done
- *Objectives* – the proportion of diabetic patients who have had their fundi/feet/blood pressure/glycated haemoglobin (HbA_{1c})/vibration sense examined during the past year

Outcome
- *Definition* – the changes in patients' health status that can be attributed to care given
- *Objectives* – level of diabetic control (HbA_{1c}, blood glucose); number of patients in practice admitted to hospital with diabetic ketosis or hypoglycaemia during a fixed period of time; number of patients developing diabetic complications over a fixed period of time; level of patient satisfaction with the service provided

Specific audit objectives and the measures of quality of care

Specific, clearly defined audit objectives should be identified for each chosen subject, focusing on important aspects of patient care. What the practice wants to know about the quality of patient care, and why, enables appropriate measures of quality to be developed and helps in the interpretation of audit results and in the implementation of action to achieve improvement. In working out the objectives for audit, it helps to think in terms of the structure, process and outcomes of patient care, and then to define the objectives accordingly. For example, an audit of the care of patients with diabetes could look at the aspects of care outlined in Box 10.3.

Whether standards or audit criteria should be set before or after finding out what is happening is sometimes a matter for debate. Setting audit criteria is extremely important, particularly if data collection, or finding out, is to be done by an audit 'assistant'. These are effectively the measures of the quality of care. An audit criterion is a statement of how a component of patient care is to be measured. This is not to be confused with a standard of care, which specifies how patient care should be provided, and is based on knowledge of external evidence and professional experience (e.g. clinical guidelines). Audit criteria depend on audit objectives and methods for data collection, specifying what and how patient care should be audited, and should be based on up-to-date knowledge, judgement, experience and best available external evidence.

Ideally, each audit criterion (standard or performance indicator) should address four main areas:

1 Which aspect of care is being audited (structure, process or outcome)? What is the minimum essential evidence on which to base a judgement of performance, or to set a 'standard'?

Example: Suppose that the practice is interested in secondary prevention for ischaemic heart disease, and wants to find out whether patients with established ischaemic heart disease have been prescribed prophylactic aspirin. Prescription of aspirin is a process measure and there is an assumption here that this process is a valid proxy for a desired outcome – reduction of future myocardial infarcts. What is the evidence to support the prophylactic prescription of aspirin for patients with angina or following a non-fatal myocardial infarct, to prevent future events (within the next 5 years)? Should all patients be prescribed prophylactic aspirin if they suffer with angina or after a non-fatal myocardial infarct?

2 In what percentage of cases would you expect clinicians to conform with the performance target (indicator) or standard?

Example: At first sight, this should be 100%. However, as the evidence for prophylactic aspirin was only published in the last year, would you expect all your patients with angina and after non-fatal infarcts to be on aspirin? Would you set a target for a specific percentage, or would you prefer to find out what percentage of patients are on aspirin first?

3 What are the known exceptions to the defined aspect of patient care under audit, and what are the clinically acceptable situations that would account for failure to conform to the set standard (performance target) (in this case, prescribing aspirin)?

Example: Patients with a known history of peptic ulcer would be an exception to being prescribed aspirin. Think of a few more.

4 There should be a clear definition of the data to be used to measure compliance with the standard. This includes definition of specific terms and numerical values, exceptions and where the data is to be found (e.g. registration database, patient records).

Example: You identify the patients with a diagnosis of ischaemic heart disease from the patient registration database. What diagnostic codes would you use for your search? How would you identify patients on prophylactic aspirin from the prescribing database? You will need to review patient records for exceptions. What would you look for? Think of some more audit questions.

Although developing audit criteria can seem laborious, time-consuming and limits the overall approach to assessing the quality of patient care, agreed audit criteria allow conclusions to be drawn from the findings that might be sufficient to support implementation of remedial action. Clear definitions for the data and where to find the information allows the audit to be performed by a non-medical 'assistant', making the exercise more cost effective. The development of audit criteria is also a learning experience for the participants.

Culture of change to improve quality of patient care

The next important step in the audit cycle is to analyse the findings from the data collected to find out if what is happening is what ought to happen in an ideal world. This completes the quality assessment process by identifying the gap between what is happening and what should be happening, but will not of itself improve the quality of patient care. To narrow this gap, it would be necessary to find out why there is a gap, what the problems might be and their causes. Decisions have to be taken about what changes are needed to improve the situation, implementing the changes, then following up with another audit after an agreed time lapse to make sure that the changes were effective. This cycle could well be repeated over several years with reviews and updating of clinical guidelines as new knowledge and technology emerge. The audit cycle could perhaps be better considered as a quality assurance spiral. The whole practice team, and GPs in particular, has to be motivated to implement changes to improve the quality of care, however that might be measured.

In our example of aspirin-prescribing for ischaemic heart disease, suppose that you found that 60% of patients with known ischaemic heart disease were having repeat prescriptions of aspirin. This is presented to the practice team at the monthly clinical meeting. You also tell the practice that having reviewed the records of patients not on aspirin, you found that some were discharged from hospital without aspirin, but had not been picked up when they came to surgery for review. Some had had a long history of angina and had never been put on aspirin, despite several 'medication reviews' for repeat prescribing. A tiny number were allergic to aspirin, a few had a history of peptic ulcer. A few more were of working age and paying for their prescriptions and, on enquiry, their 'regular' doctor remembers that they were buying their aspirins over the counter, but this had not been recorded anywhere in the notes.

The practice team (including the receptionists who process repeat prescriptions) agree that there needs to be change to improve the prophylactic prescribing of aspirin for patients with ischaemic heart disease. They decide that excluding aspirin allergy and peptic ulcer disease, they want to increase the rate to 90% over the next 6 months.

What are the clinical and organisational issues related to implementing the changes necessary for improving aspirin prescribing? Who are the members of the team that would be involved? What opportunities are there for prescribing for patients at risk not on aspirin? Should there be a practice protocol for this change? How would you remind everyone concerned about prescribing aspirin? How would you monitor the effects? How would you evaluate the effectiveness of prophylactic aspirin?

This audit subject could be discussed with your fellow registrars on the half-day release course, or could be for real in your practice. Try to work out solutions to the problems that you expect and try to think of some other issues that may be specific to your practice.

Acceptance of peer appraisal

The kind of numerical audit described above should be complemented by case reviews of variation in practice that give rise to increasing patient risk, or worse, adverse events. For example, if the diabetic audit in Box 10.3 showed that two patients were admitted to hospital twice with ketoacidosis in the preceding year, would the GP accept peer appraisal of his or her clinical practice and agree to change practice so that diabetics with persistently raised HbA_{1C} have their diet or their oral hypoglycaemic or insulin regime reviewed? What if the GP practises alone? These and other related issues fit in with the concept of clinical governance, and will be further discussed under clinical risk management.

Confidentiality in audit

Both the patients whose care is being evaluated and the doctors (and other health professionals) whose behaviour and judgement are being assessed are entitled to confidentiality. A fundamental principle in audit is the respect for privacy and confidentiality. It might be wise to agree a confidentiality policy before embarking on audit. There might, however, be occasion to 'blow the whistle' in the case of an underperforming doctor. When is this justified? When does the judgement or behaviour of a colleague become such a high risk to patient care that this can no longer be tolerated? How does one deal with it effectively? When clinically adverse events occur, whose responsibility is it in terms of shared governance? These issues will be further discussed in Chapter 11.

Research in practice

Practice-based research can often fill in the 'gaps' in evidence and could emerge through audit. For example, after doing the aspirin audit, you might wonder 'is aspirin the best prophylactic treatment for *my* ischaemic heart disease population, given our particular social and demographic characteristics, which are very different from the sample in the research?' In other words, you are asking 'how many deaths did the prescription of aspirin to *my* ischaemic heart disease population prevent in the ensuing 5 years?', which is a research question.

With so much to do in just a few months, most registrars find it difficult to carry out a research project during the training year in general practice. It would be much easier if the practice was already taking part in a research project, or if training in research methods were readily accessible. Carrying out a piece of audit is now required for summative assessment and the practical principles have much in common with research. Learning to critically appraise research evidence, useful for the written MRCGP examination, is also a good way to learn about research method. There are many good courses on how to do research that you might want to sign up to. The Royal College of General Practitioners ran a series of Master Classes in Primary Care Research and published workbooks developed from these (Carter et al 2000); there is also an accompanying CD-ROM. The series addresses quantitative and qualitative research methods, some statistical concepts, ethical considerations, how to apply for funding and more.

The intention in this section is not to provide a condensed account of research methods (see Chapter 9 or Armstrong et al 2000), but to reflect on some issues that relate to the appropriateness and feasibility of research in practice. Curiosity and commitment are the first prerequisites for anyone embarking on research. The purpose of the research must be to improve diagnostic, therapeutic and prophylactic procedures, and to contribute to a better understanding of the natural history and causes of diseases.

Often, practices are invited to collaborate in randomised controlled trials and multicentre research using an experimental design with their patients. For example, the Medical Research Council has a General Practice Research Framework of participating practices that could be recruited for multicentre studies. Local research networks could also give support, training and a forum for sharing ideas and findings from research initiatives.

Most of the interventions and procedures concerned in clinical research could involve hazard to some extent. This is understandable in a trial of alternative or new treatments but it could also be argued that some questions asked in a survey could provoke anxiety and distress. The issues to reflect upon here would be whether the practice is well organised for conducting research, and the ethical issues relating to patients as subjects for research.

Practice organisation for research

Most practice patient registers are now computerised. Suppose that you agree to recruit patients for a large, multicentre trial of alternative treatments for hypertension. The inclusion criteria are that the patients should be male or female, aged between 40 and 64, with established hypertension and on medication to control blood pressure. The exclusion criteria are that they must not be diabetic or have diagnosed ischaemic health disease. The project is funded adequately to reimburse the practice for time spent on identifying the patients eligible for the trial, and for recruiting the patients.

Reflect upon whether your patient database is good enough to support a search for suitable subjects for the study. The age and sex of the population should be no problem. How would you identify patients with hypertension?

- Are patients coded for hypertension? How reliable is the coding?
- Are blood pressure recordings accurately and reliably coded?
- Is it possible to identify hypertensive patients from their medication?
- How accurate and reliable are the diagnoses for diabetes and ischaemic heart disease?

- Do the practice staffing resources allow for the time and effort required for identifying patients for the study?

In a nutshell, is the practice database good enough and is there someone who can do the necessary search without disrupting the normal administrative routine of the practice? On the other hand, to maintain an accurate and up-to-date patient database that could double as a disease register to support audit (and items of service claims and other performance targets) will need designated staff, and such a database would be perfectly adequate for research.

What are the benefits of taking part in this research?

For the patients, some of those volunteering to take part might gain immediate benefit from having the new and better treatment, screening and surveillance, but, on the other hand, this might be hazardous. In the long term, they will have helped to find a more effective treatment for high blood pressure.

For the practice there might be a 'feel-good' factor in making a contribution towards finding a better treatment for hypertension and for adding to an understanding about the natural history of hypertension. At a more practical level, the accuracy of the practice register for recording hypertension, diabetes and ischaemic heart disease might be improved. There will be an increase in workload for whoever looks after the patient register. The amount will depend on how good the register is to begin with.

Patient consent to take part in practice research

Before approaching your patients you should first be convinced that the experimental intervention offers some hope of re-establishing health or alleviating suffering. The potential benefits, hazards and discomforts of the new treatment must be weighed against the advantages of the best, currently available treatment. You should only agree to collaborate if you believe that the benefits outweigh the risks. The eligible patients can then be invited to volunteer for the experiment.

Informed consent can be said to be in two parts. The information given on which the patient has to make a choice must be comprehensive, so that the patient is fully informed of the risks and benefits of the experimental treatment and of the experimental procedures. The information must also be comprehensible, compatible with the patients' educational and cultural background with time for questions and consideration. The second part of informed consent – the consent (or permission to be entered into the trial) – must be given entirely voluntarily, free from coercion. For example, a patient might fear that their normal treatment would be compromised if they refuse permission, and payment of 'expenses' could be seen as inducement. It has been said that doctors do not pay enough attention to the issues relating to informed consent. Do reflect on these, as the issues around consent to participate in research are generalisable to consent to other forms of treatment.

Confidentiality is another important part of research ethics. The confidentiality of records that could identify individuals must be protected, respecting the privacy and confidentiality rules in accordance with regulations (for example the Data Protection Act).

> **L** Even if you do not yet anticipate conducting formal research in your own practice, it might help to foster an enquiring habit of mind to keep notes of questions that occur to you in the daily course of your work and that would lend themselves to a piece of research, for example 'Why do some patients present frequently with minor illness and others very seldom?', or 'What would happen to the workload if the surgery was routinely open on Sundays?'

Summary

- Successful audit and research begins with a good, well-defined question.

- A good question is interesting, important and relevant, and answerable within a reasonable period of time.

- The main areas of general practice audit and research are clinical, epidemiological, operational and behavioural.

- Audit aims to improve the quality of patient care by comparing what is being done against a standard and remedying identified deficiencies. Audit does not have to be complicated to improve care.

> **L** The MRCGP examination does not currently require evidence of candidates' ability personally to conduct an audit. Why do you think this is?

References

Armstrong D, Armstrong M, Grace G 2000 Research methods and audit in general practice. Oxford General Practice Series, Oxford

Carter Y, Shaw S, Thomas C (eds) 2000 Master classes in primary care research. The Royal College of General Practitioners, London

Further reading

Baker R 1988 Practice assessment and quality of care. Occasional paper no. 39. The Royal College of General Practitioners, London

Gray J, Majeed A, Kerry S, Rowlands G 2000 Identifying patients with ischaemic heart disease in general practice: cross-sectional study of paper and computerised medical records. British Medical Journal 321:548–550

Howie J G R 1989 Research in general practice, 2nd edn. Chapman & Hall, London

Hughes J, Humphrey C 1990 Medical audit in general practice: a practical guide to the literature. Kings Fund Centre for Health Services Development, London

Irvine D, Irvine S (eds) 1991 Making sense of audit. Radcliffe Medical Press, Oxford

Lawrence M, Schofield T (eds) 1993 Medical audit in primary health care. Oxford General Practice Series, Oxford.

Morrell D 1988 Epidemiology in general practice. Oxford University Press, Oxford

Sackett DL, Haynes RB, Guyatt GH, Tugwell P 1991 Clinical epidemiology: a basic science for clinical medicine. Little, Brown & Co, Boston, MA

11 Clinical risk management

Hilary Scott

Clinical care is a risky business; although people and systems can combine to bring great benefits to patients and practitioners, the same combinations can lead to damage to both. Although first thoughts might spring to prescribing errors or missed diagnoses, other consequences of poorly managed risk in general practice include trips and falls. All practitioners and healthcare organisations have a duty to recognise the risks inherent in providing care and to take steps to minimise their effect – risk management.

Risk management can be defined as 'a means of reducing the risk of adverse events occurring in organisations by systematically assessing and reviewing them, and then seeking ways to prevent their occurrence. Clinical risk management takes place in a clinical setting' (NHSE 1998).

Risk management measures should, therefore, identify sources of risk, keep the likelihood of error to a minimum, and recover and learn from error quickly.

Recognising that risk cannot be eliminated, but that it *can* be managed, is crucial. Policies or procedures will not, of themselves, provide a risk-free experience for patients and practitioners. This idea itself might be part of the reason why, until relatively recently, the whole issue has had a fairly low profile. If we cannot make care safe, an argument ran, should we invest a great deal in trying? This approach ended for a number of reasons. The introduction of clinical governance arrangements (see Chapter 8) for the NHS made it very clear that quality in care was the responsibility of individual practitioners, managers and the organisations in which they worked (trusts and practices alike). Several very worrying incidents in NHS organisations (e.g. the results of inquiries into paediatric cardiac surgery at the Bristol Royal Infirmary and the retention of organs at Alder Hey Hospital) illustrated what could happen when that responsibility was not taken seriously. The Chief Medical Officer's report *An organisation with a memory* (Department of Health 2000) highlighted the fact that the NHS collected little information about adverse incidents and had few means of doing anything about those it did know about. And much of the (largely US- and acute-care-based) research on safety and risk in health care began to draw the attention of larger numbers of practitioners in the UK.

This led to a new focus on risk in health care at national and local levels and renewed postgraduate and continuing education efforts. Thinking and language are beginning to shift again. Some are suggesting that 'risk' is thought to imply that there are identifiable acts of omission or commission that can be regulated in some way. Using the term 'vulnerabilities', it is thought, might make it easier to appreciate that the issue has softer edges and involves greater complexity than might appear at first sight.

> **L** It is unlikely that questions about real, as opposed to fictional, high-profile incidents will be asked in the written paper. However, oral examiners may well ask about real high-profile events that have recently attracted widespread attention (e.g. Bristol, Alder Hey), and will expect candidates to have some thought-through opinions about what has gone wrong, how it may have happened, and what action should be taken.

A practice that takes clinical risk management seriously

Practices that take risk management seriously have distinguishing features. Most obvious will be a set of processes and procedures that describe how problems are picked up in the practice, how they are reported and recorded, and how the analysis of the information recorded leads to action that minimises the likelihood of a recurrence. Notes about the most important of these appear below. More subtle signs might also be present: staff who listen for, and to, concerns about the care they provide; staff who apologise for and learn from mistakes; practices that accept fault when appropriate and offer timely and appropriate redress – in all, practices that are developing a 'just' culture (this is possibly a more reasonable term than a 'blame-free' culture).

On arrival – induction

The practice will have an induction session for all its new staff. Aside from introducing new colleagues to the practice's staff and systems, the session covers what staff should do if something goes wrong or worries them at work, the way complaints are dealt with, and who is responsible for dealing with both. If there is no such session, formal or informal, registrars should ask these questions anyway.

Procedures and protocols

Commonly understood and recognised areas of high risk for patients (and staff) will be reflected in up-to-date guidance and protocols covering those areas of practice and work. They might cover clinical matters (e.g. diagnosis of meningitis in children), responsibilities for the health and safety of staff (e.g. transferring patients to and from a couch) and practice management issues (e.g. following up diagnostic test results that are not received within an expected period of time). Where appropriate, procedures and protocols will also be described in information that is specifically designed for and available to patients and staff.

The structure, coverage and use of clinical guidelines and protocols are discussed in Chapter 9. The same approach and care will be applied to health and safety at work guidance, which will cover all aspects of practice work, from disposing of sharps and other clinical waste to dealing with distressed and demanding patients and maintaining contact with practitioners when they are visiting patients at home.

It is sometimes said that the discussion about what goes into a protocol or procedure is the most valuable part of the whole process of introducing one in the first place. Thereafter, some procedure manuals and written guidance just gather dust. As a consequence they are outdated and of little use when a situation arises that leads someone to look for guidance.

In this area, three things will distinguish a practice that takes risk management seriously from others. First, it will have a rolling programme for reviewing all procedures and protocols, with those that cover known high risks to patients and practitioners reviewed more regularly than others. Second, the discriminating and thoughtful use of procedures and protocols is promoted through discussion, education and by example. Adherence to protocol is no substitute for making balanced judgements and no defence if there is a complaint. When the patient goes 'off protocol', so must practitioners. Third, there will be a named and senior member of the practice staff responsible for reviewing current procedures and protocols and ensuring others are developed, as needed.

When something goes wrong

Reporting errors and problems, and acting upon them are essential features of risk management systems. A practice will have recognisable methods for identifying, recording, analysing and responding to errors and problems.

> **L** Dealing with a complaint, grievance or clinical error is a common scenario in the written paper. As well as your theoretical answers, based on risk management protocols, examiners will expect you to show a sense of realism and to be aware of any dangers that, paradoxically, could arise from an overprominent risk management culture.

Identifying problems – error reporting

National systems   Three reporting systems are 'national' and readily recognised. The first – the Yellow Card Scheme – allows practitioners to report unexpected and/or adverse drug reactions to the Committee on Safety of Medicines/Medicines Control Agency; the second requires equipment failures to be reported to the Medical Devices Agency (see Useful contacts section at the end of this chapter), even where operator error is involved; the third are the reports required by the Health and Safety Executive (and the law) where an accident involves serious injury or death, or leads to more than 3 days away from work for a member of staff. Practices should have clear guidance on what an individual should do when one of these situations arises.

Local systems   A practice-based error reporting system will provide the opportunity to address serious and/or recurring errors through changes in practice, additional training and learning in general. The safety literature emphasises the value of anonymity when reporting errors, and this forms the basis for the national reporting system that will be introduced in the NHS during 2002 by the newly created National Patient Safety Agency (see Useful contacts section). The aim is to encourage reporting so that trends can be analysed and used to back action at a national level. An anonymous system might not, however, be a very practical proposition for most general practices, even if anonymised information is then reported to and aggregated at Primary Care Trust level. The practice will have adopted a procedure that has the greatest chance of success in its own circumstances.

A practice-based system will, again, be the responsibility of a named and senior member of staff. Information about reported error will be recorded and include the circumstances, time of day, involvement of all members of staff and the consequences of the error. The incident will be examined so that the root cause of the error can be identified, and action in response agreed upon. Aside from agreeing upon changes in practice or procedure, or specific training, the practice will also have to decide whether and how any patients who might have been affected by the error are told about it. For example, if there has been no harm to an individual, the practice might refer to the events in a section of its Annual Report about action taken following an error. A patient directly affected by an error should always be told about the examination of the error and action taken as a result. Some could argue that this might encourage complaint and even litigation; others would say that complete openness about errors and the response to them can only promote trust between people and the practitioners who care for them.

A serious incident procedure

The practice should have a separate procedure for dealing with a serious incident. This will usually be to do with an unexpected adverse event that involves serious distress or harm to a patient or a member of staff. Although many such incidents can be dealt with as reported errors, others might require, for example, the additional support of an expert from outside the practice, or someone with an independent view. Very occasionally an incident might be a matter for the police. The purpose of a serious incident procedure is, once again, to examine the events so that their root cause can be identified, and action in response agreed upon. A person suffering an adverse effect will be involved in any investigation and be kept informed of its conclusions and consequent action.

For the most part, serious incidents can be investigated and followed up 'in house'. A serious incident procedure should, however, lead a practice to ask whether a person who suffered an adverse effect could reasonably be expected to have confidence in a totally 'in-house' process, in the circumstances. A different and, perhaps, more transparent process might be required.

L As an exercise, consider what risk management procedures would have needed to be in place to have contained the damage done by the murderer Dr Harold Shipman, or by a sexually predatory doctor.

A complaints procedure

The Terms of Service for GPs require them to have a system for dealing with complaints. This means that all practices are required to have a practice-based complaints procedure, which is part of the NHS complaints procedure (at the time of writing, this procedure was under review; a revised procedure, which might change the way the second (review) stage is managed, should be in place by April 2003). The practice-based procedure represents the first stage of the national procedure: it is referred to as local resolution. Essentially, patients will be aware of, and have easy access to, a person to whom they can address a complaint and from whom they can expect a full and appropriate response within a reasonable period of time. A particular problem for the complaints process in family health services is the difficulty some patients have in approaching a practice with a complaint. They fear they will have to 'confront' the person caring for them, someone with whom they might have consulted for some time. They might also fear that complaining will result in them being removed from the practice's list: something that concerns patients more than is properly recognised by some practitioners. Complaining via a hospital complaints manager seems much less stressful by comparison. The practice-based procedure will try to address these issues in its literature and in the way staff are trained and supported when dealing with complainants and, indeed, potential complainants. Once more, a named and senior member of the practice will have responsibility for managing the complaints process and signing off responses to complainants.

If a complainant is not satisfied by the response given at the end of local resolution, he or she can ask the Primary Care Trust to set up an

Independent Review Panel to look at the complaint again. If the Primary Care Trust, having consulted with an independent person (drawn from a panel of people appointed by the Secretary of State), declines to set up a panel and the complainant is unhappy with the reasons given for this, he or she can ask the Health Service Ombudsman, who is independent of the NHS, to investigate (see www.ombudsman.org.uk for examples of the Ombudsman's work). A complainant can also approach the Ombudsman if an Independent Panel reviews the complaint but the complainant is not satisfied with the Panel's response. The Ombudsman will usually consider an investigation only if both the first and second stages of the NHS complaints procedure – local resolution and the review stage – have been completed.

A well-managed local complaints procedure gives patients confidence that problems they raise will be treated seriously and sympathetically, and provides the practice with valuable information about a different category of 'things that go wrong'. The category might overlap with 'errors' and 'serious incidents' but will be made up, principally, of other types of adverse events. There are, in fact, comparatively few complaints made about health services; but the sources of complaint are well known. Many involve incomplete explanations about care, failures in communication between professionals and patients and their families, and failures in communication between professionals. Systematic survey of complaints can lead to changes in organisational and personal practice, and to reduced numbers of complaints.

The practice should offer practical advice and support in dealing with a complaint. There will be guidance that reminds all staff that most complainants want only:

- to be taken seriously
- a clear and full explanation of the events complained about
- an apology, if one is needed
- action to prevent the same thing happening to anyone else
- a full response within a reasonable period of time.

If a complaint is made about you, you should:

- try not to take it personally; complaints are often not a personal matter at all
- take it seriously
- try to recall everything you can about the events complained about and write it down. If you are not sure what the complaint is about, ask the senior partner or the practice manager
- decide whether you would like the advice of your professional body.

> **L** It is important to know the main formal and legally sanctioned complaints and grievance machinery, not least because it is easy to draft multiple choice questions based on it!

Clinical risk management – information for learning

A practice might have all the processes and procedures mentioned above documented and in place, and still mismanage clinical risk. The problems arise when the information derived from one process is kept separate from that of another. Trends and effective responses to them are best identified when information from each of the procedures is linked with that from other sources, including clinical audit and performance indicators. Although most of the risk management literature is to do with care in hospital, areas of high clinical risk in primary care are well recognised (i.e. prescribing error, diagnosis and communication).

> **L** You might think that the most common or most important mistakes in practice are errors of clinical judgement, rather than system errors or breakdowns of communication. What factors make some individual doctors more prone to make clinical mistakes than others? Apart from protocol-based approaches to risk management, what can be done to identify, contain and correct such factors?

The practice's clinical governance arrangements should be based on drawing together information from these and other sources (internal and external) and providing further links, to education and research activity, and to opportunities for reflection on the issues arising from them all. This can only promote regular discussion of clinical risk management at this and the most senior levels in the practice, and clear accountability for action arising from those discussions.

Points for reflection

1 Much has been spoken and written about the 'blame and shame' culture in the NHS and about efforts to create blame-free organisations as the basis for identifying and learning from mistakes. For some, however, 'blame-free' sounds rather like 'accountability-free' and they speak of 'just' and not 'blame-free' cultures. Is this just semantics?

2 If you have ever been complained about, or made a complaint yourself (to any sort of service organisation), or supported a friend or colleague in such circumstances:

- Was there anything that particularly disturbed you about the experience?
- Was there anything that particularly impressed you about the way the organisation(s) involved handled the complaint?
- Is there any practice or procedure you would recommend to someone running a practice-based complaints procedure (or warn them about!)?

3 Variability in practice can be seen as both a liability and a benefit. On the one hand, failing to follow what is accepted as reasonable practice can lead to disaster. On the other hand, variability is thought of as a sign of an essential human characteristic '... human variability in the shape of compensations and adaptations to changing events represents one of the system's most important safeguards' (Reason 2000). How do you know you strike the right balance?

4 'Errors are…consequences rather than causes' (Reason 2000). If more people thought of error like this, would error reporting be more commonplace?

5 Complaints, error reporting systems and serious incident investigations point to the same problems occurring over and over again. Poor communications, poor support and supervision for junior staff, prescribing errors. Why are some lessons so hard to learn?

6 The table below describes some real incidents. Rank them in an order that you think runs from the most serious to the least. There is no more information about them: sometimes, this is all the information you may have to base decisions about immediately required action.

How serious?

	Scenario	Rank
1	Blood sampling by a practice nurse leaves a patient with extensive bruising and swelling, from wrist to shoulder.	
2	A patient calls the practice twice, complaining of vomiting and constipation. Telephone advice is given on both occasions to maintain fluids. Within 24 h the patient has died following gastrointestinal haemorrhage.	
3	A patient walks into the surgery complaining of a 'tight chest' and breathlessness on exertion. The GP cannot fit him in and he is seen by the Practice Nurse. He tells her he has been diagnosed with asthma. She prescribes an inhaler. Within 48 h the patient has died following a myocardial infarction (heart attack).	
4	A patient complains about increasing head pain, lethargy and loss of appetite. The GP diagnoses stress-related syndrome. During a particularly distressing episode his wife calls an ambulance. Referred for CT from A&E, a tumour was found from which he died 2 months later.	
5	A woman attends the surgery as a temporary resident. She has had diarrhoea and vomiting for 3 days, saw her own GP 2 days ago who diagnosed gastritis, but now feels even worse. She tells the GP she has type 2 diabetes. The GP confirms the diagnosis of gastritis. A week later the woman has been admitted to hospital with diabetic ketoacidosis and has died.	
6	A member of staff reports scalding himself while unloading the autoclave. He is off sick for a week.	
7	One of the District Nurses is reported as having a batch of 10 blank prescriptions signed by one of the partners in a practice.	
8	A patient whose anticoagulant therapy is being monitored in the practice is now also being treated for depression. She walks into the practice complaining of joint pain and bruising. The drug prescribed (Nefazodone) has interacted with the warfarin.	

Ask another doctor to do the same: better still, ask a nurse and a manager colleague to join you. The rankings are unlikely to be the same. Talk with your colleagues about the reasons why they ranked the incidents as they did, and the basis for the differences in view between you.

Summary
- All practitioners and healthcare organisations have a duty to recognise the risks inherent in providing care and to take steps to minimise their effect (i.e. managing those risks).

- Risk management can be defined as a means of reducing the risk of adverse events occurring in organisations by systematically assessing and reviewing them, and then seeking ways to prevent their occurrence. Clinical risk management takes place in a clinical setting.

- Practices that take risk management seriously have distinguishing features: most obvious will be a set of processes and procedures that describe how problems are picked up in the practice, how they are reported, recorded and responded to; more subtle signs will be to do with practice culture.

- Effective responses to risk are best identified when information from several sources informs discussion and education, often as part of practice clinical governance arrangements.

References

Department of Health 2000 An organisation with a memory. HMSO, London
NHSE 1998 Clinical governance in North Thames. Department of Public Health, NHSE, Leeds
Reason J 2000 Human error: models and management. British Medical Journal 320:768–770

Further reading

Department of Health 2001 Building a safer NHS. HMSO, London
Institute of Medicine 2000 To err is human: building a safer health system. National Academy Press, Washington DC
Public Inquiry into Children's Heart Surgery at the Bristol Royal Infirmary 1984–1995. In: Learning from Bristol. HMSO, London (Cmnd 5207)
Reason JT 1990 Human error. Cambridge University Press, New York

Royal Liverpool Children's Inquiry. Report. HMSO, London
Vincent CA 1995 Clinical risk management. BMA Publications, London, pp 31–54
Wilson T, Sheikh A 2002 Enhancing public safety in primary care. British Medical Journal 324:584–587

Useful contacts

Health Service Ombudsman
www.ombudsman.org.uk

Medical Devices Agency
www.medical-devices.gov.uk

Medicines Control Agency
www.mca.gov.uk

National Patient Safety Agency
www.npsa.org.uk

12 Continuing professional development and revalidation

Jeannette Naish

At the time of writing, the legislative framework and mechanisms for revalidation of all doctors including GPs are still under development. There has been wide consultation between the General Medical Council (GMC) and all relevant professional bodies about the procedures and resources that are needed to implement a reliable and workable revalidation programme. The principle that all doctors need periodic assessment, probably in 5-year cycles, to ensure that they continue to be fit to practise has, however, been firmly adopted. Fortunately, most doctors perform well most of the time, but in recent years there has been an unfortunate series of serious medial failures and scandals, including the infamous case of the GP Harold Shipman. The move to revalidation must be seen in this light, and in terms of the general culture change in modern society whereby government and public quite properly expect greater accountability in all walks of life.

L Continuing professional development and revalidation are important topics within the RCGP and therefore for the membership exam, not least because the RCGP is itself a significant player in their planning and implementation. As an aspiring member, you will be expected to have well-informed opinions about these and other issues of particular concern to the RCGP.

The GMC registers a doctor at the completion of basic professional training as fit to practise within the defined parameters of good medical practice (GMC 2001a) which includes clinical care, relations with colleagues, probity and personal health. The duties of a doctor registered with the GMC are also clearly outlined (see Useful contacts section at the end of this chapter). The Royal College of General Practitioners (RCGP) and the General Practitioners Committee of the British Medical Association (BMA) have also produced a document to try to define what good medical practice for general practitioners might be (RCGP 2001). The proposal regularly to revalidate doctors' fitness to practise aims to give the public confidence that their doctors provide safe and high standards of care. This concept fits with those of clinical governance (see Chapter 8), which seeks to nurture a culture of excellence. Continuing professional development (CPD) then becomes a part of this process to demonstrate a commitment to lifelong learning to ensure that the doctor remains fit to practise.

> **L** You should be familiar with *Good Medical Practice* and other high-profile material published by the GMC, the BMA, the RCGP and the Department of Health.

The revalidation process

Following the consultation process, the GMC agreed a revalidation model in May 2001. The process will normally have three stages:

- Stage 1 – collecting information and yearly appraisal
- Stage 2 – 5-yearly assessment
- Stage 3 – the GMC decision.

Stage 1 – collecting information and yearly appraisal

All GPs will have to collect a portfolio of information to demonstrate how they are achieving the standards laid out in *Good Medical Practice* (GMC 2001a), otherwise known as 'profiling the doctor's performance', in which audit will have a central role. They will be required to participate in annual peer appraisal, which gives an opportunity, together with a trained appraiser who is also a GP, to reflect on what they have achieved and whether they have attained the standards in *Good Medical Practice*. The appraisal process also aims to identify the strengths and weaknesses of the appraisee's performance over the preceding year, to identify learning needs and to plan personal and practice professional development for the ensuing year.

The portfolio

Details of what is expected in the portfolio, or folder of information about the doctor's performance, are laid out in the GMC publication on revalidation, *Revalidating Doctors* (GMC 2001b). Where doctors work in clinical teams, the information needed for their revalidation should be generated in the course of their everyday work. The information in the portfolio could be thought of as a series of folders that cover the components of *Good Medical Practice* and will be the basis for appraisal and subsequently revalidation. It would be important to get this right from the beginning, and the GMC will work with the organisations responsible for delivering training to ensure that the requirements for revalidation are embedded in vocational training for general practice. To be revalidated, each doctor will need to demonstrate that she or he is fit to practise in line with the GMC's guidance in *Good Medical Practice* (GMC 2001a), which relates to seven broad headings:

1 good professional practice
2 maintaining good medical practice
3 relationships with patients
4 working with colleagues
5 teaching and training
6 health
7 probity.

The folder will therefore:

■ Contain the doctor's relevant personal details, such as year of qualification, place of qualification, higher degrees and so on.
■ Describe what the doctor does – surgery hours, appointment systems, accessibility, out-of-hours arrangements; a description of work outside the practice, the places where the doctor has worked and, where relevant, the locum agencies with which he or she has been employed, and a description of the field or fields of practice in which the doctor has worked during the revalidation period.
■ Contain information to demonstrate the doctor's performance and describe the steps the doctor is taking to stay up-to-date and to develop professionally. This information should be collected against each of the general headings in *Good Medical Practice* (GMC 2001a).

Information about performance should come from a wide range of sources including, wherever possible, the doctor, his or her patients, the doctor's colleagues and the doctor's managers. Doctors will be expected to provide information on:

■ Their pattern of performance – details of a piece of audit (see Chapter 10) performed and written up by the doctor.
■ Continuing professional development – courses attended, the aims and objectives for attendance and impact on clinical practice, whether these meet patient needs and what the doctor's future learning needs might be.
■ Critical incidents (see below) – a critical incident (or adverse event) review within the framework of risk management. The Medical Defence Union has devised a good clinical risk management pack (see Chapter 11).
■ Patient complaints and compliments – procedures for handling complaints, whether these are audited and what, if any, lessons are learned and procedures for improvement implemented (see Chapter 11).

■ The results of any external assessments, such as Royal College or Deanery accreditation for training.

> **L** What do you know about the latest arrangements for implementing appraisal in your own locality? What problems do you envisage, and how might they be overcome?

Example of use of a critical incident   Consider the following case illustration, when there had been an incident with an aggressive patient in the reception area.

Case illustration

> The patient seemed very reasonable to begin with when asking for an appointment to see Dr A, who is 'his' doctor. The receptionist, who was also busy on the telephone, told the patient that Dr A was not available that day, but Dr B was, and that she would book the patient with Dr B. The patient insisted that he must see Dr A. The receptionist then asked if it was urgent and had to be the same day. The patient became very aggressive, shouting at the receptionist that she was not a doctor and had no right to judge the seriousness or urgency of his problem, that Dr A was dealing with the problem and would be the best person to sort things out. The receptionist told the patient that the practice rule is that if the patient's doctor of choice is not available, he must see the next available one, unless the problem is 'urgent', in which case they could be fitted in as an 'extra'. Further harsh words ensued, followed by a formal written complaint from the patient a few days later about the impossibility of accessing his doctor of choice.

How would you review this incident, and what lessons might be learned?

■ Is there a record of patient complaints and/or aggressive incidents kept in the surgery?
■ If there is a record, would a review or audit of the types of complaints and incidents be useful?
■ What is the appointment system? Are there enough appointments to meet the patients' needs? Have appointments been audited?

Think of some other (clinical) topics (apart from patient complaints and aggressive incidents) that you might use to demonstrate how the doctor and the practice performs. What opportunities might there be to reflect on the doctor's and the practice's developmental/learning needs?

Annual appraisals   It is proposed that periodic revalidation is backed up with annual reviews of the doctor's practice. This will consist of annual peer appraisal with the aim of reviewing the information in the portfolio to see what the appraisee has achieved and whether they have met the standards in *Good Medical Practice* (GMC 2001a). During the process, gaps and learning needs should be identified and an action plan should be formulated to address the need. At the end of this process, the appraisee and appraiser have to confirm that the information has been reviewed regularly and an action plan agreed. This confirmation might take the form of a signed statement agreed during an annual appraisal by appraiser and appraisee.

Remember that:

■ The purpose of appraisal is formative – to support doctors in maintaining and improving their professional performance.

■ The appraisal process should include another registered medical practitioner who is professionally accountable to the GMC, in addition to any contractual accountability.

■ Appraisal should include (but need not be confined to) a review of a doctor's revalidation folder. Gaps in the information should be identified and filled before the end of the revalidation cycle so that the assessment is as straightforward as possible.

■ Appraisal should identify likely difficulties with a doctor's practice that need to be addressed in the course of the run-up to the assessment at the end of the revalidation cycle. There should be no surprises at the end of the cycle.

■ In identifying any difficulties, the appraisal should highlight where they are caused or exacerbated by practice conditions, equipment, or levels of staffing.

■ Appraisal should ensure that the description of what the doctor does is accurate and that the information about his or her fitness to practise is sufficient.

■ The appraiser should be able to arrange any developmental or remedial action that is deemed necessary as a result of the appraisal.

■ The detail of the appraisal discussion should be confidential.

■ One outcome of each annual appraisal should be a statement, which will be placed in the revalidation folder, confirming that a satisfactory appraisal process has taken place and identifying any developmental needs. The agreed statement should be signed and dated by the doctor and the appraiser.

■ Where, exceptionally, the review of information reveals danger to patients that cannot be resolved by an agreed plan of action, the appraiser must explain to the doctor that, in accordance with every doctor's professional obligation to protect patients, he or she will be taking whatever steps are necessary to safeguard patients. These might include the kinds of remedial measures proposed in *Supporting Doctors, Protecting Patients* (Chief Medical Officer 1999).

Stage 1 is essentially formative, with self-reporting of activities to demonstrate performance followed by an annual review. This links in with Stage 2, which is summative. Within the context of lifelong learning and CPD, the appraisal is an excellent opportunity to take time out for reflection about *what* you are doing, *how well* you are doing it and *where* you would like to go for both personal interest and practice development. A number of publications seek to give guidance on how to prepare for Stage 1 of which *Professional Development: A Guide for General Practice* (While & Attwood 2000) is one.

> **Consider...**
>
> ■ Think about what qualities you would value in your appraiser.
> ■ Prepare for a mutual appraisal session with a colleague as practice.
> ■ Discuss with your colleagues in a small group: the process, how you felt, what went well and what could be better, from the perspective of appraiser and appraisee.

Stage 2 – 5-yearly assessment

Stage 2 is the summative part of revalidation. It is the responsibility of individual doctors to submit their portfolio for assessment. A revalidation group made up of members of the public and doctors will assess the information in the portfolio every 5 years and recommend to the GMC whether the doctor should be allowed to continue to practise. The composition and procedures for appointment of the revalidation group(s) are still under discussion at time of writing. Whatever the outcome of consultation, the revalidation group is expected to make unambiguous recommendations. Doctors will be either recommended for revalidation or referred for the GMC to review their registration.

Stage 3 – The GMC decision

On the certification of the revalidation group that the doctor has demonstrated fitness to continue to practise, the GMC will usually renew the doctor's registration. If the group does not believe that the doctor has demonstrated fitness to practise then the GMC will investigate the case further using their 'fitness to practise' procedures (Chief Medical Officer 1999). Doctors who, after consideration by the GMC, are found fit to practise will be revalidated. Those who are not found fit to practise will either have their entry on the register erased or suspended, or will have their registration made subject to conditions. Sanctions such as retraining or working under supervision might be imposed.

Summary

■ Following a period of wide consultation, the GMC agreed a revalidation model in May 2001, in a 5-yearly cycle. Three stages are proposed:

Stage 1 – A folder of information describing what the doctor does and how well the doctor does it. This will be regularly reviewed – annual appraisal will fulfil this in many sectors.

Stage 2 – Periodic revalidation. A recommendation by a group of medical and lay people that the doctor remains fit to practise, or that the doctor's registration should be reviewed by the GMC. This will probably take place every 5 years.

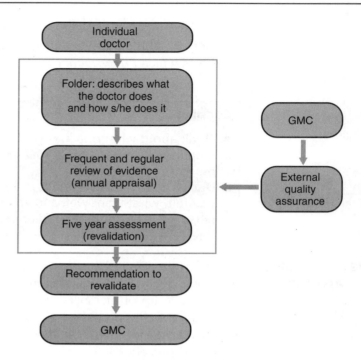

Figure 12.1
The revalidation process.

Stage 3 – Action by the GMC. In the majority of cases, revalidation of the doctor's register entry will take place. In a minority, detailed investigation under the GMC fitness to practise procedures will occur, which can lead to restrictions upon practice, suspension, or erasure.

■ In essence, after the initial full registration of a doctor by the GMC as being fit to practise, all doctors will be required to go through a process to demonstrate continued fitness to practise every 5 years to gain revalidation of this registration (Fig. 12.1).

L   How do you think continuing membership of the RCGP could be linked in with the appraisal process and the longer-term 5-yearly revalidation process?

References

Chief Medical Officer 1999 Supporting doctors, protecting patients. Department of Health, London. Online. Available: www.doh.gov.uk/cmoconsult

GMC 2001a Good medical practice. Online. Available: www.gmc-uk.org

GMC 2001b Revalidating doctors. GMC, London

RCGP 2001 Good medical practice for general practitioners. Online. Available: www.rcgp.org.uk

While R, Attwood M 2000 Professional development: a guide for general practitioners. Blackwell Science, Oxford

Useful contacts

Blackwell Scientific Publishers
www.medirect.com

Department of Health
www.doh.gov.uk

General Medical Council
www.gmc-uk.org

Royal College of General Practitioners
www.rcgp.org.uk

SECTION 4

Ethics and law in practice

13 Ethics and clinical practice

Margaret Lloyd

At the heart of clinical practice is the consultation between patient and doctor. It has been said that every clinical encounter involves an ethical (moral) decision. But what is an 'ethical' decision? We could say that it is doing the 'right thing' – but what is that and how do we decide what to do? First of all, think about the following case studies.

L Doctors at the start of their careers might not yet have encountered or recognised significant ethical dimensions in their daily practice. Examiners, on the other hand, being older, will have done so, and they like to ask questions in this field. You will almost certainly get an 'ethical' question in the orals, and it is likely there will be an ethical component to at least one written question.

Case study 1
Mr F, who is depressed

> Mr F has suffered from depression and anxiety for many years. Three months ago he started a new job. He consults you because he is feeling depressed again and attributes this to stress at work. He asks you for a medical certificate but asks you not to mention depression because he is afraid that this will jeopardise his job. What would you do and how would you justify your decision?

Case study 2
Mrs S, who has multiple sclerosis

> Mrs S is 52 years old and divorced with one son who is a student. She has had multiple sclerosis for many years and is now severely disabled and lives in a residential home. She has frequent chest infections and has asked you not to prescribe antibiotics for her next infection because she wants to die. What would be your response? How would you justify your decision?

Case study 3
Mr and Mrs N, undergoing IVF treatment

> Mr and Mrs N have been having investigations for infertility and have been offered in vitro fertilisation (IVF) treatment by a private hospital. They cannot afford the cost of the drugs and ask you to prescribe them on an NHS prescription. You know that this may restrict your prescribing of some drugs for other patients. What would you do and how would you justify your decision?

In each of these scenarios think about what you would do and what guides your decision making. You might have said that:

- Your decision was based on your own moral code; your set of moral values influenced by family, cultural and religious factors. For example, some people would never accede to the request by Mrs S because they believe, perhaps on religious grounds, in the absolute sanctity of life.
- You acted according to what you intuitively felt was right at the time. This might be your approach when dealing with Mr F.
- You were guided by your knowledge of medical ethics, the law and professional codes of practice.

It is likely that all of these influenced, to a lesser or greater extent, your decision making. A systematic review of research studies, which looked at the way in which general practitioners make ethical decisions, found that

> **L** The experience of MRCGP examiners is that candidates often find it hard to make the connection between theoretical awareness of ethical principles and their application in real life. Particularly in the orals, the emphasis will be on your ability to make (and to justify) a decision when confronted with a moral dilemma. Answers such as, 'I would ask one of the partners' or 'I would phone my defence organisation' do not impress!

the majority used 'inconsistent, individualistic methods of decision making without evidence of specific models or criteria' (Rogers 1997). But what are the moral theories or moral principles that can be used as a framework for making and justifying difficult ethical decisions? In this chapter we can look at them only briefly but if this kindles your interest to know more, you will find suggested further reading at the end of the chapter.

Moral theories

Utilitarianism

This theory, introduced by Jeremy Bentham and developed by John Stuart Mill, holds that it is the consequences of an action that determine whether the action is morally right or wrong. Another way of putting this is that 'the end justifies the means'. Therefore a utilitarian would say that killing was morally wrong, not because it is wrong in itself but because of the consequences, such as the cutting short of the person's life and the effect of their death on others. Another way of expressing the central tenet of utilitarianism is that the morally right decision is the one that produces the 'the greatest good for the greatest number'. This has the most obvious application for us when we consider the allocation of limited resources within the NHS. Would you use it to resolve the dilemma posed by the request of Mr and Mrs N for expensive IVF drugs?

Duty-based theories

The German philosopher, Immanuel Kant, believed that our actions must be determined by what we consider to be our moral duty, irrespective of the consequences of that action. For example, a person who holds this belief would say killing is always wrong in itself, not just because of the bad effects. Kant defined the supreme moral law as 'do as you would be done by' and held that people should always be treated as ends in themselves, never as the means to an end.

Duties and rights are the two sides of the same coin. We often claim to have certain rights. A person such as Mrs S might claim to have a right to decide how and when she should die. Mr and Mrs N could claim a right to free health care, including the right to receive expensive drugs. But what is a right?

A right is a justified claim that requires action or restraint from others. In other words, if you have a right to something, this implies that another person has a duty to fulfil that right. For example a person's right to life means that others have a duty not to kill them. This is an example of a negative right (a right not to be killed); other rights are positive, for example a right to education or health care. Some rights are enshrined in law, for example patients have a right to care from a general practitioner under the National Health Service Act of 1977.

Making an assertion about your rights does not necessarily establish that you ought to have that right and the rights of one person or group could conflict with another person's right. It therefore follows that not all rights and their corresponding duties are absolute. For example, patients generally have a right to confidentiality but there are times when a doctor must waive that right in the public good.

Virtue ethics   Virtue ethics places emphasis on personal qualities such as compassion and honesty rather than on utility or duty. It can be traced back to Aristotle, who believed that the person who acted virtuously was more likely to flourish than the person who was less virtuous. In summary, this theory holds that an action is right if it is what a person with a virtuous character would do in similar circumstances. This raises the question of who defines the qualities of a virtuous doctor. The application of virtue ethics to ethical dilemmas within medicine is relatively recent and is being developed (Toon 1999).

The four principles   The four principles discussed below form a useful framework for analysing ethical dilemmas. They were introduced by Beauchamp and Childress (1994) in the USA and further developed by Ranaan Gillon (1995) in the UK:

Respect for autonomy   'Autonomy' literally means 'self rule'; that is, a person who is competent to do so must be allowed to decide what is done to him- or herself, and others have a duty to respect that right. This raises the question of how we decide whether a person is autonomous and who makes the decision? Also, conflicts can arise if respecting the autonomy of one person threatens the autonomy of others. Respecting the autonomy of patients is expressed practically in obtaining their consent to an intervention, and in maintaining confidentiality.

There is now an increasing emphasis on patients being involved in making decisions about their management. This is in stark contrast to the days when paternalism ruled and the doctor always 'knew best' and acted accordingly. Our duty as doctors is to help patients to exercise their autonomy by providing the information and support to enable them to do this. However, some patients want decisions to be made on their behalf and to do so is also respecting their autonomy, although it is important not to use this argument to justify unwarranted paternalism.

Beneficence   This means acting in such a way that benefits a patient, that is, 'doing good'. It would seem to be the most straightforward of the principles but raises the question of who decides what is 'good' for the patient?

Non-maleficence   The importance of not causing harm to patients is a fundamental principle of healthcare practice. It must be balanced by our wish to do good. An example of this potential conflict of principles is raised by screening programmes, such as breast screening by mammography. The finding of an abnormality on a woman's mammogram, which, on further investigation proves to be of no serious significance, has not benefited the woman and could have caused her considerable anxiety and harm. But is this balanced by the overall reduction in deaths from breast cancer, assuming that this can be attributed to population screening?

Justice

There are three forms of justice in the context of health care:

1 distributive justice – ensuring that there is fairness in the distribution of resources (this will be discussed in more detail at the end of this chapter)
2 rights based justice – justice in respecting people's rights
3 legal justice – respecting morally acceptable laws.

The four principles are often referred to 'prima facie principles', meaning that they are binding unless they conflict with another principle. If this happens then a decision must be made 'in the best interests of the patient'. For example, in deciding your response to Mrs S's request to withhold antibiotics, you would have to balance your respect for her autonomy with your duty to 'do good' and not to harm her.

In the following sections we shall see how these moral theories and principles can help us when we are faced by difficult ethical (i.e. moral) decisions.

Decisions at the end of life

Helping patients to die 'a good death' is an important part of a general practitioner's role. The term 'euthanasia' is derived from the Greek 'eu' meaning 'well' or 'easily' and 'thanatos' meaning 'death'. In other words, euthanasia means an easy or good death and it is unfortunate that it has come to be associated with the hastening of death by medical means. It is used in a number of ways and it is important to be clear about these (Box 13.1).

Box 13.1
Euthanasia

- **Active euthanasia** – a positive action to end life (e.g. an injection of a lethal substance or disconnection of a ventilator).
- **Passive euthanasia** – doing nothing to save a person's life when that life might have been saved (e.g. deciding not to prescribe antibiotics for a terminally ill patient).

But the terms active and passive euthanasia are ambiguous and are best avoided.

- **Voluntary euthanasia** – ending a person's life at his or her request. This is illegal in the UK but has recently been legalised in the Netherlands. Doctors there can end the life of a terminally ill patient at the patient's request, but must follow strict guidelines.
- **Assisted suicide** – a form of voluntary euthanasia – giving a person the means to end his or her own life at his or her request (e.g. prescribing a large number of sedatives).
- **Involuntary euthanasia** – ending the life of a person who has not requested it.

The care of the dying patient often demands much of those involved and can include making difficult ethical decisions. These will be discussed in the context of the clinical scenario about Mrs S at the beginning of the chapter and two further cases.

Case study 4
Mrs V, is it morally permissible to withhold treatment?

Mrs V, who is 85, has cerebral vascular disease and has become progressively demented. She has recently had a number of strokes, which have left her with a dense right hemiplegia. She has recurrent chest and urinary infections. You are called to see her again and you diagnose pneumonia. You wonder if it is appropriate to prescribe another course of antibiotics. What would you do and how would you justify your decision?

Case study 5
Mr T, is it permissible to hasten death at the person's request?

Mr T has prostate cancer with widespread bony metastases. You recognise that he is terminally ill and that he knows this. He is in severe pain, which is barely controlled by opiates. He asks you to 'spare him the suffering by hastening the end'. How would you respond to his request and how would you justify your response?

These scenarios raise some key questions about the care of the dying. First, is 'doing nothing' (i.e. withholding treatment such as antibiotics from Mrs V or from Mrs S) morally different from doing something active to hasten death, as in Mr T's case? Does it make a difference that Mrs S has asked you to withhold treatment? Although you might feel intuitively that there is a moral difference and that doing something active is morally questionable, most philosophers argue that there is no moral difference between causing death by not doing something (i.e. an omission) and causing death by a positive act. The doctor's overriding duty is to relieve the person's suffering – to 'do good' – and this could justify both withholding treatment and hastening death by active means.

The second question concerns whether or not a person, such as Mr T, has the right to determine the manner of his or her death. This is a matter of current interest with the legalisation of strictly controlled voluntary euthanasia in the Netherlands and Switzerland. However, in the UK it remains illegal to carry out 'active euthanasia' by giving, for example, an injection of a lethal substance (such as potassium chloride) but what about a dose of opiates that will relieve pain but which you know is likely to cause respiratory depression and death?

Does a person have a right to request euthanasia? Most GPs have experienced this request and the subsequent dilemma. Many would argue that a request such as Mr T's should not arise if there is adequate palliative care for the patient. However, patients do ask doctors to relieve them of their suffering by hastening their death and such requests raise some important questions. It could be argued that you should respect Mr T's autonomy and therefore his wish to die:

- What is your duty as his doctor? This must be to prevent suffering but is it to preserve life at all cost?
- Is this benefiting the patient (beneficence) or doing harm (maleficence)?

The doctrine of double effect

This doctrine or principle, recognised by theologians and the law, permits an action that might have two effects, one that is considered 'good' and one considered 'bad'. The intention of the action must be to produce a good effect, although the possibility of a bad effect might be foreseen. For example, giving Mr T a large dose of opiates would relieve his pain (one effect considered 'good') but might lead to his death, a second effect that you did not intend, although you might have foreseen it.

The slippery slope argument

This is often used in discussions about euthanasia. People argue that allowing some actions will lead to the adoption of less desirable or even illegal actions. For example, allowing voluntary euthanasia, even under strict controls, would eventually lead to the 'killing on medical grounds' of groups such as the old and mentally ill. The slippery slope argument is also used in discussion of other ethical dilemmas but is usually not a valid argument.

Decisions at the beginning of life

Pregnancy and birth are usually happy events. However, in some situations difficult moral decisions have to be faced, more so recently because of the technological advances in reproductive biology. This section concentrates on issues raised by the termination of pregnancy.

Termination of pregnancy

Dealing with requests by patients for termination of pregnancy under the 1967 Abortion Act is now part of routine practice for the majority of practitioners. So much so that it is easy to lose sight of the moral issues involved in the abortion debate. At the extremes of the debate are those who believe in the absolute sanctity of life and think that abortion is always morally wrong – they are often referred to as the pro-life lobby. At the other extreme are those who believe that the woman has the right to choose whether or not to proceed with a pregnancy – the pro-choice lobby. The majority of doctors occupy an intermediate position along this spectrum and believe that there are situations when abortion is morally justifiable and that each woman should be treated as an individual case. It is important to look critically at your own position on abortion. Here are three case scenarios to think about.

Case study 6
Mrs J

Mrs J comes to see you for the first time when she is 12 weeks pregnant. She tells you that her pregnancy is unplanned and that she has felt very stressed since finding out. She wants a termination because she must continue to work. This is in order to pay off the large debts that have enabled her and her husband to furnish the luxury house they recently bought. She tells you 'I have a right to have a termination because it's my body'.

Case study 7
Ms D

Ms D lives with her unemployed partner and three children. The youngest is 2 years old and Ms D has only just fully recovered from postnatal depression. She is very upset to find that she is pregnant again and asks for a termination saying that she wouldn't be able to cope with another baby. A scan shows that she is 14 weeks pregnant.

Case study 8
Mrs K

Mrs K is a 40-year-old woman in her first pregnancy. A scan at 16 weeks' gestation shows that the fetus has anencephaly. This is explained to Mrs K and she is offered termination of pregnancy, which she refuses on the grounds that her baby has the right to life and that abortion would be 'murder'.

In all of these cases termination of pregnancy could be carried out legally but what moral issues are raised? Mrs J's pregnancy is socially inconvenient and she clearly thinks that she has the right to decide what happens to her pregnancy. But does she have such a right and does a doctor have a corresponding duty to agree to arrange a termination for her? Many would feel that social inconvenience is not a morally acceptable reason for terminating her pregnancy. Although by agreeing to her request you would be respecting her autonomy, some would argue that her right to choose should be balanced against the right to life of her fetus. This argument revolves around the question of whether a fetus should be regarded as a person who has rights, a non-person or a potential person, and is the subject of much philosophical debate. An appropriate position, which accords with the law, is that the protection given to a fetus is dependent on its degree of maturity, that a fetus of 8 weeks should have less protection than one of 18 weeks.

It is likely that you would feel more sympathy with Ms D's request and would have no problem in justifying your support for her to have her pregnancy terminated.

Ms K's decision must be respected and it would be important to give her as much support as possible throughout her pregnancy and afterwards. This scenario raises the difficult question of why abortion up to 24 weeks is within the law (the fetus has no legal status) but the killing of a baby 24 minutes after birth is classed as murder.

Remember!
- Your duty is to give a woman all the necessary information and support her in her decision making.
- Think about your own values. If you are totally opposed to abortion you should refer the woman to a colleague who holds different views.

Truth telling

Telling a patient 'the truth' is usually seen in the context of the doctor delivering bad news, for example telling a patient that they have a life-threatening illness. But patients also need accurate information if they are to give informed consent to an intervention; they need to know the benefits and risks of the procedure. Patients have a right to know the truth and doctors have a duty to provide it.

However, truth telling is much more than giving patients accurate information about their illness or an intervention; it is recognising and helping patients to exercise their autonomy, to share in the decision-making process about their management. It is being sensitive to the needs of patients – how much information do they want and when should it be given? There is considerable evidence that patients want to be told the truth about their illness and prognosis. Gone are the days of the doctor's paternalism when it was considered that patients should be protected from the truth of having a life-threatening illness. Of course, telling the truth is not easy and demands a sensitive approach and good communication skills. There are occasions when it could be that telling the truth causes a person more harm than good, but these situations are probably rare. The withholding of the truth might destroy the trust not only between individual patients and their doctor, but also between the public and the medical profession.

Truth telling tests the balance between respect for autonomy and paternalism, between beneficence and non-maleficence. Honesty is one of the characteristics of the virtuous person.

Resource allocation

How should limited healthcare resources be allocated? On what basis should choices between patients be made? These are difficult questions but ones that GP practitioners have to face. There are no easy answers, although in the UK, the National Institute of Clinical Excellence (NICE) is contributing to decision making by issuing evidence-based guidelines, which might be contentious, on the cost-effectiveness of interventions.

First of all, consider the case of Mr and Mrs N who ask you to prescribe expensive drugs in their attempts to conceive by IVF. Would you prescribe for them and how would you justify your decision? Some points you might consider and discuss are:

- You have a duty of care to them – a duty of beneficence. But does this include helping them to conceive by artificial means? Do individuals have a right to procreate if they wish?

- Would you be depriving other patients of treatment, assuming that you had a limited drug budget? Do you not have a duty to them?
- Should you adopt the utilitarian principle of using resources to obtain the greatest benefit for the greatest number of patients?
- What emphasis should you place on the evidence of the cost-effectiveness of a treatment?

Difficult decisions might also have to be made between patients requiring the same treatment that is strictly limited by cost or availability such as organs for transplantation. What criteria should be used to decide which patients should receive treatment? These could include:

- random allocation
- 'first come, first served'
- age – the young should be preferred to older patients because they have a greater life expectancy
- family responsibilities – the father of three young children over the middle-aged bachelor
- social worth – the Mayor over the homeless tramp
- merit – the person's contribution to society; the consultant cardiac surgeon to be preferred over the unemployed labourer
- the probability of medical success
- those who have the greatest medical need.

There is no generally agreed framework that is morally acceptable to all. Many would agree that the last criterion (i.e. the patient who is judged to have the greatest medical need) would be the fairest way of allocating scarce resources and that interventions should be, as far as possible, evidence based.

Summary

- Decision making in the majority of consultations has an ethical (moral) component.

- You should always be prepared to justify the decision you make.

- An understanding of moral theories and principles provides a framework for decision making.

L The answer to many ethical questions is 'It all depends'. For exam purposes, you need to be aware of what your 'bottom line' principles are, or where, if pushed, you would 'draw a line in the sand'. The examiners might start with a relatively easy question such as 'Would you accept a bottle of wine from a grateful patient?'; they might then 'up the ante' by continuing, 'What if it was a £5 note? £100? A valuable legacy?'

L You might try keeping an 'ethical issues log' during some of your routine surgeries, in which you note ethical issues such as 'How truthful should I be?', or 'In what ways does the cost of a drug or a patient's circumstances affect my prescribing?'. You might not meet many extreme examples, but hard cases make bad law. Nevertheless, you will begin to familiarise yourself with your own ethical assumptions, and how you would justify them.

References

Beauchamp TL, Childress JF 1994 Principles of medical ethics, 4th edn. Oxford University Press, Oxford

Gillon R 1995 Philosophical medical ethics. John Wiley, Chichester

Rogers WA 1997 A systematic review of empirical research into ethics in general practice. British Journal of General Practice 47:733–737

Toon P 1999 Towards a philosophy of general practice: a study of the virtuous practitioner. RCGP Occasional paper no. 78. RCGP, London

Further reading

British Medical Association 1993 Medical ethics today: its practice and philosophy. BMA Publishing, London

Campbell A, Gillett G, Jones G 2001 Medical ethics. Oxford University Press, Oxford

Hope T, Savulescu J, Hendrick J 2003 Medical ethics and law. Churchill Livingstone, Edinburgh

Orme Smith A, Spicer J 2001 Ethics in general practice. Radcliffe Medical Press, Abingdon, Oxfordshire

14 Professional codes, the law and clinical practice: consent and duty of care

Margaret Lloyd

In Chapter 13 we looked at the moral theories and principles that underpin and guide our clinical practice. These find practical expression in the law and the professional codes of conduct for doctors, and will be discussed in this chapter. We shall start with some general points about the law and professional codes and then deal with the important topics of consent to treatment, medical negligence and dealing with complaints.

Clinical practice and the law

As citizens we are all bound by laws of various kinds. They are laid down by Acts of Parliament (statute law) or by the courts (case or common law).

Statute law

Examples of statute law that are relevant to general practice include the Abortion Act, the Notification of Infectious Diseases Act and the Mental Health Act. The Human Rights Act 1998 came into force in 2000 and its main provisions, which are applicable to medical practice, include respect for human dignity and a person's right to life and privacy. The impact of this Act has yet to be established.

A general practitioner's Terms of Service were laid down by Act of Parliament as part of the National Health Service Act of 1977 and the Health Act of 1999, which allowed the creation of Primary Care Trusts.

> **L** The GP's Terms of Service ('The Red Book') is arguably the most important but least read document you will encounter. Make sure you are acquainted with its main points, together with (if appropriate) the terms of your practice's PMS contract.

Case law

Case, or common, law is made by the courts. The lowest court dealing with civil cases (which includes all cases of medical negligence) are county courts and coroners courts and the highest is the House of Lords. When a court is considering a case they are bound by previous rulings that have been made in similar cases in a higher court. For example, the action brought by Mrs Gillick about the prescribing of oral contraceptives to girls under the age of 16 was eventually heard by the House of Lords, whose ruling is now binding on all courts (*Gillick* v. *West Norfolk and Wisbech Area Health Authority* 1986). Courts cannot override statutes, although they can seek to interpret a statute when it does not exactly fit a case under consideration.

Ethics and the law

On the whole, behaviour defined as legal in a society will also be considered to be moral, and illegal behaviour considered immoral.

An interesting question is whether a doctor can behave morally but illegally? An example of an act that is legal but would conflict with the moral principles of some doctors is the referral of a patient for termination of pregnancy under the terms of the Abortion Act. Conversely, a doctor who signs a medical certificate 'lassitude' for a patient suffering from depression, such as Mr F in Chapter 13 (p. 160) who is afraid that his job would be threatened if his employer knew the diagnosis, could be said to be acting against the law but morally because he was acting in the patient's interests.

As we shall see later in this chapter, fundamental concepts of clinical practice, such as consent to treatment, are firmly grounded in the law, either by statute or by case law.

Professional codes of practice

The first code of conduct was the Hippocratic Oath on which all codes for healthcare professionals are based. A modern version of the oath was written by Dr Howard Spiteri:

> *The physician shall selflessly practise medicine for the sole benefit of the patient and shall avoid causing him harm. He shall do so with respect, integrity and compassion without any form of prejudice.*

Codes are needed to protect patients because some conduct that can harm patients might be perfectly legal (e.g. breaking a patient's confidence). In the UK, professional codes are established by the General Medical Council (GMC), which was set up by the Medical Act of 1858. Its duty is 'to protect patients and to guide doctors' and its functions are summarised in Box 14.1.

In 1985, the Professional Conduct Committee of the GMC began to concern itself with the standards of care provided by doctors as well as with their personal conduct. In 1995 the GMC published the first edition of *Good Medical Practice,* which placed patients' needs at the centre of the picture. Fourteen duties of a doctor are listed preceded by the statement (GMC 1995):

Patients must be able to trust doctors with their lives and well-being. To justify that trust, we as a profession have a duty to maintain a good standard of practice and care and to show respect for human life.

L You should be familiar with all 'high profile' documents published by the GMC, especially *Duties of a Doctor and Good Medical Practice* – not least because the MRCGP exam syllabus is based on the latter!

Box 14.1
Functions of the General Medical Council

- Setting and assuring educational standards for medical schools
- Keeping the up-to-date register of qualified doctors
- Issuing guidance about the standards expected of registered doctors
- Dealing with doctors whose fitness to practise is questioned
- Reaccreditation of doctors

Consent and withdrawal of consent

A sound doctor–patient relationship is built on a trusting partnership, where patient and doctor are partners in the decision making. This means that information should be shared with the patient and his or her consent to treatment obtained. However, this is not always a straightforward process and it is important to have a firm grasp of the professional codes and the law concerning consent to treatment and refusal of treatment. But first of all consider the following case studies and think how you might manage these situations.

Case study 1
Mr M and his demented mother

Mr M calls you to see his 82-year-old mother who has Alzheimer's disease and peripheral vascular disease. When you examine her you find that she has the signs of a femoral artery occlusion with early signs of gangrene in her foot, and you decide to refer her to hospital. Mr M is worried about his mother being able be give consent to surgery and asks you if he can sign the consent form. How would you reply?

Case study 2
Mr G, who refuses treatment because he wants to try natural remedies

> Mr G is 32 and has stage 1 testicular cancer. The consultant has advised chemotherapy but Mr G has refused this, and all other treatment, saying that he believes that a herbal remedy will cure his cancer. He has defaulted from all his hospital appointments. His wife comes to see you to ask you to persuade him to have chemotherapy. How would you manage this consultation?
>
> The following month you see Mr G because he has developed a painful shoulder after putting up shelves in his kitchen. Would you raise the issue of his refusal of treatment with him? If so, how would you do this?

Case study 3
Jenny M, aged 15, who gives consent for her operation?

> Jenny has had ulcerative colitis for several years and her last episode was so severe that the consultant has advised her parents that she should have an ileostomy. Who can give consent?

Valid consent

Always obtain a patient's consent to a procedure

This a moral and legal obligation. By obtaining consent you are respecting the person's autonomy. Patients have a right to determine what is done to them and doctors must respect this right. In law, failure to obtain consent could result in the patient bringing a claim of battery against the doctor, even if the failure to gain consent has not caused the patient any harm; touching the patient without consent is considered harmful in itself.

This means that the patient must:

- Be competent to give consent. All persons aged 16 years and over are assumed to have the capacity to give consent unless you can demonstrate otherwise. If you judge that the patient is not competent to give consent you must be prepared to justify your decision.
- Be fully informed about the nature of the procedure, the benefits and risks and alternative treatments. Failure to provide a patient with adequate information about a procedure may result in a claim of medical negligence against the doctor. The main problem in cases of this nature is what constitutes 'appropriate information'? This point has arisen in a number of legal cases and the courts have usually decided on the basis of what most doctors would consider appropriate (i.e. the Bolam test; *Bolam* v. *Friern HMC* 1957).
- Give consent voluntarily; that is, without undue pressure from anybody else, including the healthcare professionals looking after them.

A patient can withdraw their consent

Even if the patient has signed a consent form, he or she can withdraw consent at any time, assuming that he or she is considered competent to do so.

Assessing competence

A person is judged competent if they are over 16 years and are able to:

- understand and retain the information given to them
- believe the information
- weigh up the risks and benefits to arrive at a decision.

It is important to note that a person's capacity to consent must be assessed in relation to a specific treatment. So, for example, a patient with mental health problems might be judged competent to make some healthcare decisions but not others.

In the case of Mrs M, the hospital doctor should use these criteria to decide whether or not she had the capacity to consent to the operation. Occasionally, it might be necessary to obtain independent psychiatric advice when assessing a person's competence.

In many instances patients imply their consent by their actions, for example, by laying their arm on your desk when you ask to take their blood pressure. Contrary to what is often thought, consent to an intervention can be given verbally or in writing. A signed consent form is not a legally recognised document except as evidence that consent has been obtained. However, it is wise to obtain written consent, particularly if the procedure is complex or carries significant risk of harm. When obtaining consent to a procedure, a brief description of your discussion with the patient should be recorded in the patient's notes. The Department of Health has produced guidelines and a consent form for use in hospitals (DoH 2001).

No consent by proxy

No adult can give or withhold consent on behalf of another person aged 18 or over.

This applies even if the patient lacks the mental capacity to give consent. In such a case a doctor should do what he or she considers to be in the best interests of the patient. If a patient is detained under the Mental Health Act, treatment can be given only for the mental disorder or a related physical condition.

In the case of Mrs M, her son could not sign the consent form even if she was judged to lack the capacity to give informed consent. The surgeon could operate without her consent if he considered it to be 'in the best interests of the patient'.

Emergency situations

A patient can be treated without consent in an emergency if he or she is unable to give consent, for example, if they are unconscious, emergency treatment can be given 'in the best interest of the patient'. In common law this is covered by the doctrine of necessity.

Refusal of treatment

All competent adults have the absolute right to refuse treatment. You must respect a competent patient's decision to refuse treatment, even if it seems illogical to you and even if it means that their life is threatened. The criteria for judging their competence are the same as those for deciding whether or not a patient can give consent. The most commonly quoted example of refusal of treatment is the refusal of Jehovah's Witnesses to accept blood transfusions. There have been several successful court cases in the UK and USA against doctors who have not respected their patients' decisions.

In the case of Mr T, who is a competent adult, his decision to refuse treatment must be respected. This may be a difficult situation for the doctor to handle, particularly when the patient has a life-threatening condition that has a good prognosis with conventional treatment. It would be the doctor's duty to respect the patient's decision but also to reinforce the information about the prognosis with and without treatment.

There have been cases of pregnant women refusing caesarean section, even when the life of their fetus is at risk. The latest court ruling in the UK was that a woman who is considered competent has the absolute right to refuse treatment even though this might result in her death and/or the death of the fetus. In this and all other situations when patients refuse treatment, full and accurate record keeping is essential.

If a competent person voluntarily makes an advance directive or 'living will', for example refusing resuscitation, this is legally valid and his or her wishes must be respected even if the patient subsequently becomes incompetent.

Children and adolescents

Parents, or those with parental responsibility, can give consent to treatment for their children who are under the age of 16. However, it is recognised that children can and should be involved in decisions about their treatment and can give legal consent, depending on their level of maturity. This was established in law by the House of Lords' ruling in the case brought by Mrs Gillick against her local health authority. This concerned the provision of contraceptive advice to her children under the age of 16. Lord Scarman said:

A minor — is capable of giving informed consent when he or she achieves a sufficient understanding and intelligence to enable him or her to understand fully what is proposed.

L The Gillick ruling and other landmark legal cases are a fertile source of oral questions.

The duty of the doctor is to establish whether the young person fulfils these criteria and be able to justify that decision.

Jenny could give consent if she was considered mature enough and able to fully understand the procedure and its implications. It would be more usual for her parents to give consent for the operation and to involve Jenny in the decision. If Jenny refused surgery, her parents could still give consent – a very difficult and undesirable situation.

Adolescents between the ages of 16 and 18 are legally able to give consent if they are considered competent to do so, and their consent cannot be overridden by their parents. However, parents and the courts can override refusal of treatment. In recent years there have been several cases of adolescent girls with anorexia nervosa who have refused artificial feeding but whose wishes have been overridden by the courts.

Consent for medical research

The conduct of research on human beings is governed by the Declaration of Helsinki, which stresses the importance of obtaining the fully informed consent of participants. All research projects involving patients require the approval of a local ethics committee. All committees stipulate that patients must be fully informed about the nature of the research and their consent must be given voluntarily and obtained in writing. The requirement that consent must be given voluntarily is particularly important in the context of research studies; no pressure should be put on the patient, however much you wish to recruit them to your study. It must be made clear to a patient that their refusal to participate will in no way affect the quality of the medical care they receive. The obligations on the researcher to provide the patient with information about the benefits and risks of the research are greater if the research is 'non-therapeutic', that is, it does not benefit the patient directly.

Care of the mentally ill

Dealing with patients with mental health problems raises ethical, professional and legal issues. The balance between respecting a person's autonomy, acting in the patient's best interest (beneficence) and not causing harm (non-maleficence) is often challenged in caring for patients with mental illness and learning disabilities.

Legally, patients and doctors are protected by the Mental Health Act 1983, which covers patients who have mental disorders (this includes mental illness and learning disability). Box 14.2 outlines the sections of the Act that are most applicable to the general practitioner.

Complaints and litigation

Dealing with complaints

The number of complaints by patients in increasing, although they are less likely to complain about their general practitioner than hospital doctors. The increase is a reflection of patients' increased expectations of healthcare professionals and the increasing culture of consumerism within the health service. Patients have a right to complain if they feel that they have received an inadequate service. The most frequent motive for them doing so is to seek an explanation for what went wrong and to prevent the same thing happening to someone else.

In any practice, a certain number of complaints by patients is inevitable. Some will be substantiated and some not, but all will cause anxiety and an additional work load. The key thing is the way in which they are handled within the practice. There is now an established procedure for handling complaints, which practices must follow as part of their service requirements (Box 14.3). The monitoring and handling of complaints is part of clinical governance. Investigation of complaints should be seen as an opportunity to improve the quality of services which a practice provides for its patients. Moreover, the early and sympathetic handling of a patient's complaint is less likely to leave them feeling aggrieved and resorting to legal action.

> **L** Responding to a complaint is a common scenario in the orals and written paper. The feelings of the doctor or other person complained about – guilt, anger, embarrassment, fear – are often neglected in candidates' answers.

Box 14.2
The Mental Health Act (England and Wales)

Section 2 (for assessment)

- Maximum length of detention is 28 days.
- Application by an approved social worker or nearest relative. The latter is defined as the person with whom the patient 'ordinarily resides'.
- Must be supported by two doctors, one of whom is approved under section 12 of the Act. Ideally, one should have knowledge of the patient. The time interval between the two doctors examining the patient should be no more 5 days. Form 3 to be completed.
- The patient has the right of appeal to a Mental Health Review Tribunal in the first 14 days.

Section 4 (in emergency situations)

- Maximum length of compulsory admission is 72 h.
- Patient must be admitted within 24 h or earlier of the application.
- Application by the nearest relative or an approved social worker – they must have seen the patient within the previous 24 h.
- Application supported by a doctor who has knowledge of the patient or approved under section 12 of the Act. They must have seen the patient in the previous 24 h.

Box 14.3
Procedure for handling complaints

- Every practice must identify a person responsible for receiving and investigating all complaints.
- Patients must be informed of the procedure.
- All complaints must be recorded in writing, acknowledged in writing or orally within 3 days of receipt and investigated.
- The complainant must be given a written report of the investigation within 10 days of receipt of the complaint.
- All records and relevant letters must be kept separately from the patient's records.

Medical negligence

Every doctor has a fear of being sued for negligence. In the UK and USA the number of claims against doctors is rising fast. Four billion pounds was set aside by the NHS in 2002 to cover outstanding claims; this is equivalent to 6% of the total annual NHS budget. This increase has led to the practice of what is often called defensive medicine, for example, ordering an investigation that is not indicated clinically but which is carried out 'just in case'.

In 1998 the Medical Defence Union reported that 66% of negligence claims against general practitioners were related to delays in diagnosis and 25% to prescribing errors. The great majority of negligence cases are heard in the civil courts where decisions are made 'on the balance of probabilities'. Very occasionally doctors are referred to the criminal court, where cases must be proved 'beyond reasonable doubt'.

The purpose of medical negligence actions is to obtain compensation for patients. Many claims are settled out of court and of those that reach the courts only the minority are successful. In fact, it is difficult for a patient to bring a successful claim for negligence against a doctor and the process is long and often traumatic for patient and doctor. To bring a successful claim, a patient must prove that:

- The doctor had a duty of care to them – GPs have a legal duty of care to the patients on their lists.
- The standard of care was inadequate – this raises the question of who establishes the standard of care? Who decides what the doctor should have done and therefore whether or not his actions were negligent? Traditionally this has been the medical profession on the basis of the Bolam test, which states that: 'A doctor is not negligent if he has acted in accordance with a practice accepted as proper by a responsible body of medical men skilled in that particular art'. However, in recent cases the courts have been moving away from using the Bolam test and have become more involved in deciding what the standard of care should be.
- The harm to the patient was caused by that breach of duty – this is usually the most difficult part of bringing a successful claim of negligence against a doctor. Patients must prove that but for the doctor's breach of duty (i.e. mistake) they would not have suffered the injury.

Case study 4
Dr A and Mr Y, a complaint followed by legal action

Mr Y consulted his GP, Dr A, complaining of chest pain which had started after he had done some gardening. He was worried because he had had a heart attack 3 years ago although the pain didn't feel quite the same. Dr A's surgery was running late and he didn't examine Mr Y because the pain sounded muscular in origin. Next day the practice received a letter of complaint from Mr Y saying that he had been kept waiting and had not been examined. One week later Mr Y was admitted to hospital and died the next day. Post mortem showed that he had a large anterior myocardial infarct. His widow lodged a claim of negligence against Dr A.

How would you respond to Mr A's letter of complaint? (see Box 14.3) Remember that a complaint dealt with sympathetically is less likely to lead to the patient or their relatives taking legal action.

Is Mrs A's claim of negligence likely to succeed in court? Dr A certainly had a duty of care to Mr Y as his GP. Although it could be argued that Dr A breached his duty of care by not examining Mr Y, it might be difficult to prove that this led to Mr Y's death. After all, the pain for which he consulted Dr A might have been muscular in origin, followed by an unrelated myocardial infarction the following week.

Case study 5
A 'Good Samaritan' act

> One evening you are out with friends when one of them draws your attention to a man who has collapsed outside a bar. A crowd is gathering. What would you do?

One option would be to walk by and do nothing, but if you were a GP principal in your practice area this would be breaching your duty of care even if the person was not on your list. If it happened outside your area you would not be legally obliged to attend to the person, but in France you would be flouting the law and liable to a jail term. However, you might consider that you had a moral duty and the GMC would certainly expect you to offer help. In its booklet *Good Medical Practice* (GMC 2001) the GMC states that you should offer to anyone at risk 'treatment you could reasonably provide'. Once you did this, and said that you were a doctor, then you have a duty of care to the person and could possibly be sued if things go wrong, although this would be a rare occurrence. Fortunately, the medical protection organisations in the UK now cover doctors for Good Samaritan acts.

Summary

- All doctors are bound by professional codes of practice and by the law, as well as by their own moral code.

- A knowledge of the basic principles and facts concerning consent to treatment and refusal of treatment is essential.

- Complaints made by patients must be dealt with according to a standard procedure.

- All doctors have a legal duty of care to their patients and failure to discharge this duty could result in a claim of medical negligence.

- Poor communication between doctor and patient is often the cause of complaints and litigation.

References

Bolam v. *Friern HMC* 1957 2 All ER 118

Department of Health (DoH) 2001 Reference guide to consent for examination or treatment. DoH, London

General Medical Council (GMC) 2001 Good medical practice. GMC, London

Gillick v. *West Norfolk and Wisbech AHA* 1986 AC 112

Further reading

Leung W-C 2000 Law for doctors. Blackwell Science, Oxford

Mason JK, McCall-Smith RA 1994 Law and medical ethics. Butterworths, London

15 Confidentiality and access to records

Margaret Lloyd

Whatever I see or hear, professionally or privately, which ought not to be divulged, I will keep secret and tell no one (the Hippocratic Oath).

Patients have a right to expect that information about them will be held in confidence by their doctors. Confidentiality is central to trust between doctors and patients (General Medical Council 2000).

The confidential nature of the doctor–patient relationship has been one of the cornerstones of good medical practice since the time of Hippocrates. Although this is so, and we recognise the confidential nature of what a patient tells us, there are times when the handling of confidential information presents us with a dilemma. In this chapter we shall look at three aspects of confidentiality and then apply the principles to some clinical scenarios. First of all we shall briefly discuss:

■ the ethical and legal basis of confidentiality
■ the General Medical Council's guidelines
■ when disclosure of information can be justified.

The ethical and legal aspects of confidentiality

Respect for a person's autonomy is a key aspect of good medical practice. The information a patient gives to a doctor is owned by that person and he or she has the right to say if and when it can be shared with others. As doctors we have a duty of confidentiality to a patient. However, this duty can occasionally conflict with our responsibility to society, as we shall see later in the chapter.

Trust is the essential basis of the doctor–patient relationship. Patients put their trust in a doctor, to whom they might divulge information they do not wish to be disclosed to anybody else. If this trust is not respected, patients are unlikely to divulge sensitive information that could be important in their diagnosis and management.

Confidentiality and the law

There is no overarching law governing confidentiality in the UK, unlike in France and Belgium where a breach of confidence is a criminal act. In the UK, the doctor's duty of confidentiality is not absolute and the attitude of the courts has been based on a few individual cases (i.e. common law). As a general rule, the courts rely heavily on the code of practice set out by the General Medical Council. However, doctors do have a statutory duty (i.e. laid down by Act of Parliament) to disclose information under certain circumstances.

Confidentiality and the General Medical Council

The General Medical Council, in its latest guidance document, has listed seven principles of confidentiality which should guide our practice (GMC 2000). These are summarised in Box 15.1.

Box 15.1
GMC's guidance on confidentiality

■ Patients have a right to confidentiality. Their consent must be sought for disclosure of information and the reasons and likely consequences discussed with them.
■ Information about a patient must not be disclosed to third parties, save in exceptional circumstances.
■ Health workers to whom you disclose information must understand that it is given to them in confidence, which they must respect.
■ You must be prepared to explain and justify any decision you make about withholding or disclosing confidential information.
■ Make sure that confidential information is effectively protected against improper disclosure when it is disposed of, stored, transmitted or received.

Box 15.2
When the law demands information

- Notification of births and deaths under the Birth and Death Registration Acts
- Notice of termination of pregnancy under the Abortion Act of 1967
- Treatment of drug addicts to be notified to the Home Office under the Misuse of Drugs Act (Notification of Supply to Addict) Regulations 1973
- Notification of infectious diseases (e.g. tuberculosis, food poisoning) to the district Consultant in Communicable Disease Control
- When a warrant is issued by a circuit judge under the Police and Criminal Evidence Act 1984
- When a judge in court demands information

When can information be disclosed?

Our duty of confidentiality to patients is not an absolute one and breaches of confidence can be justified under some circumstances. These include:

- When a patient consents to disclosure of information about themselves. The consent must be in writing for disclosure to a third party and you must document the consent in the patient's records.
- Disclosing information to those who need to know in order to provide the patient with appropriate care.
- When the wider public interest outweighs the duty of confidentiality.
- When the law demands it. Health professionals are obliged by Acts of Parliament to disclose some information, even if the patient objects. These are shown in Box 15.2.

Case studies

Case study 1 *Ms F and her driving licence*

Ms F has just qualified as a teacher and has recently joined your practice. She tells you that during the summer holidays she had a grand mal fit and, after investigations, was diagnosed as having idiopathic epilepsy. She asks for a repeat of her medication and questions the need for her to stop driving as she finds it difficult to get home on public transport after late evenings at school. In fact she admits that she has not informed the DVLA and has driven her car a couple of times after parent–teacher meetings.

How would you manage this consultation?

The regulations of the Driver and Vehicle Licensing Agency (DVLA) state that a person must not drive for 1 year after an epileptic fit and must inform the DVLA of the condition. After 1 year free of fits the person can reapply and a 3-year licence will usually be issued. In response to Ms F's question you should explain that:

- She has a legal duty to inform the DVLA and to stop driving.
- You will use every reasonable effort to persuade her to stop. For some patients this could include breaching confidentiality and informing their next of kin.
- If Ms F continues to drive you have a duty to breach confidentiality and inform the medical adviser at the DVLA of her condition. You must warn her that you intend to do this and then confirm it in writing.

This is an example of disclosure of information without the patient's consent when the public interest outweighs the duty of confidentiality. In the experience of most doctors it is unusual for a patient to refuse to inform the DVLA and necessitate breach of confidentiality. If the patient is not capable of understanding your advice, for example because of dementia, you should inform the DVLA immediately.

Case study 2
Mr T, who is HIV positive

> Mr T is a 35-year-old business man who frequently travels abroad. He consults you because he feels generally unwell, has a low-grade fever and lymphadenopathy. He tells you that about 2 years ago he had unprotected sex several times during a trip to Tanzania. With his agreement you arrange a series of tests including an HIV test, which proves positive. He asks you not to tell his wife who is now 8 weeks pregnant and is a patient of yours. They are planning to buy a new house and he asks you about the implications of the result for his mortgage application.
>
> How would you respond to his requests and how would you justify your response?

In general, doctors must respect the wishes of patients who do not want their HIV status to be disclosed. However, exceptions can be made on a 'need to know' basis. This could apply to other healthcare professionals and to the sexual partner of the patient. As Mrs T is a patient of the practice, you also have a duty of care to her. You would, of course, try to persuade Mr T to tell her but if he refused you would be justified in informing her, after warning Mr T of your intention to do so.

In cases of serious communicable disease the guidelines given by the GMC (1997) are that:

- You can disclose information about a patient to protect another person from risk of death or serious harm (e.g. a sexual partner or a health professional you consider to be at risk).
- You cannot disclose information to others who are not at risk of infection.
- You must always inform the patient of your intention and be prepared to justify your decision.

The relevant legal case highlighted the potential conflict between maintaining confidentiality and the public interest. The case concerned two doctors, X and Y, who were being treated in hospital for AIDS. A local newspaper was planning to publish their names and the health authority obtained an injunction preventing publication. The judged ruled that the duty of confidentiality outweighed freedom of the press.

Release of information to a third party (i.e. the mortgage company) would be a breach of confidentiality and could not be justified.

Case study 3
Stephen the arsonist

> Stephen is 21 and has been a patient of yours since childhood. He became well known to the police following a succession of petty crimes and was sent to a special boarding school. He comes to see you because he has burnt his hand and injured his foot. During the consultation he tells you that this happened when he was trying to break into the local school, which was subsequently destroyed by fire. The following week the police come to see you as part of their investigation into a spate of arson attacks in the district. They suspect Stephen and ask you if you have treated him for burns or other injuries at any time.
>
> Would you give the police the information they want. How would you justify your decision?

Legally you are not obliged to assist the police in their investigations, although of course you must not give misleading information. However, you might judge that the crime is serious enough to threaten public safety and that you would be justified in breaching Stephen's confidentiality. Would the police have access to your records? The police can obtain a warrant to gather information during their investigation of a crime. However, they cannot use a warrant to obtain confidential health records except in exceptional circumstances when they have to apply to a circuit judge for a warrant.

Case study 4
Billy and the stolen car

> Billy, aged 15, comes to the surgery covered in cuts and bruises and complaining of a painful neck. He tells you that the car he was driving crashed into a lamp-post yesterday and that one of his friends was seriously injured. He admits that they had stolen the car and that he had run away after the crash. The following day the police contact you and ask if you had treated him and had any further information about Billy.
>
> Would you give the police the information they want? How would you justify your decision?

Unlike the previous case, you are legally bound as a citizen, under the Road Traffic Act of 1988, to give the police information about the identity of a driver suspected of having committed a traffic offence. So in this case you would have to breach Billy's confidentiality and give information to the police.

Case study 5
Claire and the pill

Claire is 14 and comes to see you with her boyfriend. They have been having regular sexual intercourse and she asks you to prescribe the contraceptive pill. She and her family have been your patients for many years and you know them well. She feels it is impossible to discuss contraception with her parents and does not want her parents to know that she is on the pill.

How would you manage this consultation?

As discussed in Chapter 14, guidance about this situation comes from the Gillick case, in which the House of Lords ruled that a teenager who was judged to be mature has a right to confidentiality when the exercise of that right is in her best interest. So the onus is on the doctor to decide on the young person's maturity. If judged to be immature, the doctor can inform the parents. How can maturity be assessed? Lord Fraser ruled that a doctor can prescribe contraceptives without informing her parents if he/she is satisfied that:

- the girl understands the advice given
- she cannot be persuaded to tell her parents or allow the doctor to tell them
- she is likely to have sexual intercourse with or without contraception
- her health could suffer if she was not given contraceptives
- overall, it is in her best interests to prescribe contraceptives without the consent of her parents.

Some further questions

What can patients do if they think that confidentiality has been broken?
It is rare for patients to take legal action against a doctor for breach of confidentiality. More usually patients will lodge a complaint with the practice or the GMC. If they do decide to take legal action they might try to claim compensation for breach of contract or medical negligence.

Can a doctor be charged for maintaining confidence?
This has never been tested in law in the UK. However, in a famous case in the USA a psychologist was successfully charged by the parents of a student named Tarasoff, who was murdered by a mentally disturbed patient. The patient had told the psychologist of his intention to murder Ms Tarasoff but the psychologist had maintained confidence and had not informed the police.

Does the duty of confidentiality continue after a patient's death?
In general, the obligation to maintain confidentiality continues after a person's death. The most obvious exceptions are the requirements to sign death certificates and to provide information to the Coroner in connection with an inquest.

Beware!
- Of discussing patients in public using your mobile phone – easily done!
- Of patients seeing other people's information on your computer screen.

- Of casual conversation referring to patients in public places.
- Of leaving patients' records in accessible places (e.g. the back of your car).

Access to records

Medical records contain patients' confidential information. Over the past few years several Acts of Parliament have restricted access to personal records of all kinds and thereby have protected confidential data.

The Data Protection Act (DPA) 1998

This came into force on 1 March 2000 and replaced the 1984 Data Protection Act, which applied only to information about individuals held electronically. The new Act applies to both paper and computerised health records of living individuals. It can also be interpreted to include photographs and videos that are kept as part of a patient's record. The Act covers the acquisition, storage, use and disclosure of confidential health data. It also gives patients the right of access to the information that a practice holds about them. Generally, a patient has the right to receive a copy of their information, whenever the record was created.

A practice must register with the Data Commissioner's office, pay an annual fee and appoint a member of the practice as data controller. All information held about patients must be adequate, relevant, accurate and kept securely.

What must a patient do to access their health record?

They should make a written request for access (this can be sent by e-mail) to the data controller. They must send the required fee – £10 maximum can be charged for access to electronic records and up to a maximum of £50 for manual records. No fee is necessary if the patient just wants to view the paper records.

What must the patient be given?

Competent patients or their representatives must be given:

- a description of the information held
- all information held in the practice regardless of when the record was created
- an explanation of what it is being processed for
- a description of those to whom data may be disclosed.

The information must be given in a form that the patient understands and with an explanation if this is considered necessary. The practice must respond to the patient's request within 21 days if the information has been acquired within the previous 40 days. For records made before that, the practice must respond within 40 days. Under no circumstances must the data be amended or deleted after the request has been received.

When may access be withheld?

A patient's access to his or her notes can be withheld if you think and can justify that:

- Disclosure would be likely to cause serious harm to the patient's mental or physical health (not simple anxiety or hurt feelings).

■ Disclosing the records would mean giving information about a third party, unless the other person consents (this does not apply if the third party is a health professional involved in the care of the patient).

A patient can apply to the data controller to have factually incorrect information corrected.

The Access to Health Records Act (AHRA) 1990

This Act, which was introduced to cover manually held records, has now been largely replaced by the DPA 1998. The main exception is that access to the manual and computerised records of those who have died is covered by the AHRA, as the DPA 1998 covers only the records of living individuals. Under the AHRA, the personal representative of a patient who has died or someone who has a claim arising out of the death, can apply for access to their records. The Act only covers records made after November 1991; there is no statutory obligation to disclose records made before then. Access can be denied for reasons similar to those under the DPA.

The Access to Medical Reports Act 1988

This Act covers medical reports requested by employers or insurance companies who must:

■ inform the patient of their request in writing
■ obtain the patient's written request for their doctor to release the information
■ inform the patient that he or she has a right to see the report
■ inform the doctor that the patient wishes to see the report.

The doctor must:

■ Wait for 21 days before sending the report about a patient who has asked to see it but fails to request access.
■ Change a report at the patient's request if he or she agrees to the amendment, or append a statement of the patient's view.
■ Give a patient, who initially chose not to see the report, access to the report for up to 6 months afterwards.

Doctors can refuse a patient access to the report if they consider that it might cause the patient harm, breach the confidentiality of another person who has provided information or disclose information about a third party.

The NHS Plan 2001

As part of the NHS Plan, the government has proposed that letters between clinicians will be copied to the patient as of right and, when feasible, smart cards will be issued to patients, allowing them easier access to their health records.

Case studies

Children over the age of 16 and those under 16, if judged capable of understanding the significance of disclosure of their records (i.e. Gillick competent; *Gillick* v. *West Norfolk and Wisbech AHA* 1986), must give their own consent to disclosure. Therefore, you would have to assess

Case study 6
Mr A and his daughter's notes

> Mr A's daughter Helen is now aged 13. She has congenital heart disease and has had a series of operations to correct the defects. Mr A is worried that the family has not been given all the information about Helen's condition. You do your best to explain her condition and the treatment she has received but he is not satisfied and asks to see Helen's notes.
>
> How would you respond to his request?

if Helen was Gillick competent and, if so, ask for her consent for her father to see her notes. If you did not think that she was competent then her father would have a right of access to her records.

Case study 7
Ms C and her mother's notes

> Ms C's mother died recently from carcinoma of the colon. Ms C comes to see you expressing concern that her diagnosis was delayed because you did not refer her immediately when she presented with an episode of diarrhoea several years ago. Ms C asks to see her mother's notes.
>
> How would you handle your consultation with Ms C?

This consultation raises several issues that would need sensitive handling. Legally, under the AHRA, Ms C has a right to see her mother's medical records if they were made after November 1991. If they were made before then you would not be legally obliged to show them, although you might decide to do so. This assumes that Mrs C did not specify before her death that her notes should remain confidential.

Case study 8
Mr B, who has manic depression

> Mr B has been your patient for the last 5 years. He has had several episodes of mania during which his behaviour was very bizarre. His mood is now relatively well controlled on new medication. He has developed an intense interest in his condition and asks to see his notes.
>
> How would you respond to his request?

You would need to assess if his records contained information that might cause serious harm to his physical or mental health. This would involve you making a subjective judgement. Under the DPA you could remove sensitive information that might cause him harm from the records.

The Caldicott Report

The Caldicott Report on the Review of Patient-identifiable Information was published by the Department of Health in 1997. It focused on maintaining the confidentiality of patient records when being transferred within and between healthcare organisations. All Trusts, including Primary Care Trusts, must appoint a person as Caldicott Guardian who has the responsibility of implementing the recommendations of the report.

Summary

- A doctor has a duty not to divulge confidential information about a patient except in exceptional circumstances.

- Confidentiality can be broken if it is considered to be in the public interest to do so. You must always be prepared to justify your decision to divulge information.

- In general, patients have a right to see their medical records. Their access is governed by Acts of Parliament (i.e. statutes).

- Be aware of these rights when recording information about a patient.

L Other members of the primary care team – nurses, managers, receptionists, secretaries – also have a duty of confidentiality. What are your views on how a sensible balance can be struck between this and the need to work efficiently? Where are the chief threats to confidentiality in the day-to-day workings of a practice? How has confidentiality been affected by increasing reliance on computer-held information?

L Might there be some types of information you would choose *not* to record in the written or computer-held notes? A patient's unconventional sexuality? Marital infidelity? Crime? Are there circumstances in which you would consider removing sensitive information from the record, such as a previous termination of pregnancy, HIV risk factors or the fact that a child was adopted?
Although you will not fail the MRCGP exam if you adhere to the strictest possible interpretation of the principles set out in this chapter, most experienced doctors (and the best exam candidates) will allow that circumstances are often not black and white in real life.

But if they are not, should they be?

References

Department of Health (DoH) 1997 The Caldicott Report. DoH, London

General Medical Council 1997 Serious communicable disease. GMC, London

General Medical Council 2000 Confidentiality: protecting and providing information. GMC, London

Gillick v. *West Norfolk and Wisbech AHA* 1986 3 All ER 402–437

Further reading

Leung W-C 2000 Law for doctors. Blackwell Science, Oxford

Mason JK, McCall-Smith RA 1994 Law and medical ethics. Butterworths, London

Orme Smith A, Spicer J 2001 Ethics in general practice. Radcliffe Medical Press, Abingdon, Oxfordshire

Useful contacts

The Driving and Vehicle Licensing Agency (DVLA)
www.dvla.gov.uk/at_a_glance/content.htm

The Office of the Data Protection Commissioner
www.dataprotection.gov.uk

SECTION 5

General practice in the changing National Health Service

16 The changing National Health Service

Steve Gillam

The policy preoccupations of successive governments over the last 20 years have been consistent: containing costs and increasing efficiency, addressing variations in clinical quality, increasing professional accountability and improving access and user responsiveness. The Conservative Government introduced reforms in 1990 that concentrated on controlling costs and quality through the introduction of an internal market (NHS Executive 1994). A central policy instrument was fundholding, which capitalised on GPs' intimate knowledge of local services (derived from their traditional 'gate-keeping' function) and their financial entrepreneurialism (derived from their traditional autonomy as independent contractors).

If the previous decade had been one of unparalleled turbulence in the NHS, any expectations that the pace of change might slow with a change of government in 1997, when Labour came to power, were soon to be discarded. This chapter examines recent health policy developments from the vantage point of general practice.

L The MRCGP examination is explicitly set in the context of the UK's system of health care. Although a detailed knowledge of the historical background to the present configuration of the NHS might not be relevant to candidates who practise overseas, they should nevertheless be broadly familiar with the administrative, organisational and political systems within which British doctors operate.

The inheritance

Fundholding came to be seen as the spearhead of a 'primary care-led NHS' (NHS Executive 1994). Although its champions claimed great benefits from the scheme, the evidence to support these claims was equivocal. Most fundholding practices had produced only modest improvements, which were probably insufficient to justify their higher cost (Audit Commission 1996). Ultimately, fundholding was unsuccessful in several respects (LeGrand et al 1998). It was bureaucratic, involving high transaction costs; it was perceived as unfair – fundholders generated inequities in access to care ('two-tierism'); it was difficult to demonstrate that GPs were effective or impartial as advocates in their patients' interests; most importantly, the internal market failed to deliver anticipated efficiency gains.

Yet fundholding spawned a variety of attempts to adopt a more comprehensive and integrated approach to health care, including total purchasing, multifunds and locality commissioning (Mays et al 1999). Each in their different ways recognised a need to plan and budget for comprehensive provision, usually for populations considerably larger than the average general practice. Crucially, fundholding did entrench political support for widening the involvement of GPs in resource allocation and service planning.

The search for a better contract

General medical services (GMS) and general practice as a provider of services were left otherwise untouched by the internal market. A new contract was imposed in 1990. It provided tools to increase the accountability of GPs but failed to address deep-rooted deficits in primary care, and was criticised for its lack of local flexibility.

The *Choice and Opportunity* White Paper of 1995 (Secretaries of State for Health 1996) was in many ways a response to pressure for change from within the medical profession. The BMA was seeking to renegotiate the compulsory contractual requirement of 24-h responsibility for care and to define more tightly the nature of 'core' general medical services. Recruitment and retention of doctors was problematic and there were many indications that a growing minority of GPs were seeking salaried or alternative employment options (Lewis & Gillam 1999).

The NHS (Primary Care) Act 1997 – passed in the dying days of the Conservative Government – nevertheless marked a revolutionary change (Department of Health 1997a). The launch of Personal Medical Services (PMS) pilot schemes marked the ending of GPs' monopoly of primary medical care, with new market entrants in the shape of NHS trusts and nurses. The long-cherished national contract was no longer to apply universally with the development of alternative employment options to that of the independent GMS/general dental services (GDS) contractor. A chronology of events since April 1997 is listed in Table 16.1.

Table 16.1
Chronology of events

April 1997	*The NHS Primary Care Act* passed
May 1997	Labour Government elected
December 1997	*The New NHS: Modern, Dependable* published
April 1998	85 first-wave PMS pilots go live
June 1998	*A First Class Service* published
August 1998	Beacon practices announced
March 1999	First NHS Direct pilot evaluation reported
April 1999	Primary Care Groups (PCGs) go live
April 1999	20 first-wave walk-in centres announced
May 1999	Frank Dobson (Secretary of State for Health) announces restrictions on Viagra prescribing
October 1999	National Institute for Clinical Excellence (NICE) publishes first recommendation on Relenza
October 1999	Second-wave PMS pilots go live
November 1999	First healthy living centres launched
November 1999	*Supporting Doctors, Protecting Patients* published
December 1999	Coverage of NHS Direct extends across the country
January 2000	Harold Shipman convicted
February 2000	Commission for Health Improvement (CHI) launched
April 2000	17 first-wave Primary Care Trusts (PCTs) go live
July 2000	*The NHS Plan* published
March 2001	Tony Blair (Prime Minister) pledges £100 million to general practice: new local incentive payments
July 2001	Bristol Enquiry reported
September 2001	*Shifting the Balance of Power* published
April 2002	302 PCTs and 28 Strategic Health Authorities come into being
Wanless Report published
New GMS contract framework launched

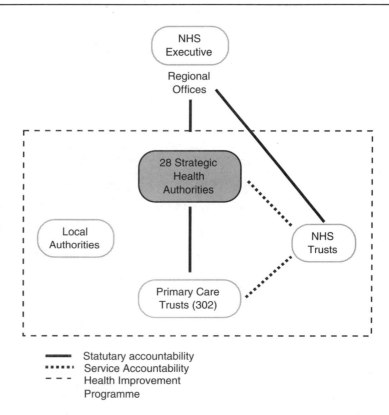

Figure 16.1
*The new NHS
structure.*

The new NHS   The publication of the Labour Government's White Paper *The new NHS:
modern, dependable* (Department of Health 1997b) formally announced
the demise of GP fundholding and the internal market. It underlined the
role of the NHS in improving health, renewed an ideological commitment
to equity in access and provision, and tackled the need to ensure quality
through clinical governance and accountability to local communities. Of
fundamental importance was the move to loosen the restrictions of the
NHS's old tripartite structure (separating general practice, hospital and
community health services) by moving towards unified budgets and
imposing a duty of partnership. The major structural change introduced
to deliver these policy goals was the formation of primary care groups
(PCGs) (Figs 16.1 and 16.2). As we have seen, that GPs would prove
efficient as stewards of the NHS was largely an article of faith.

PCGs were to undertake three principal functions on behalf of their
local populations (Department of Health 1998):

1 to improve the health of the population and address health inequalities
2 to develop primary and community health services
3 to commission a range of community and hospital services.

They brought together local providers of primary and community services under a board representing local GPs, nurses, the local community,
social services and the health authority. PCGs served populations aver-
aging around 100 000 people and were expected to evolve over time

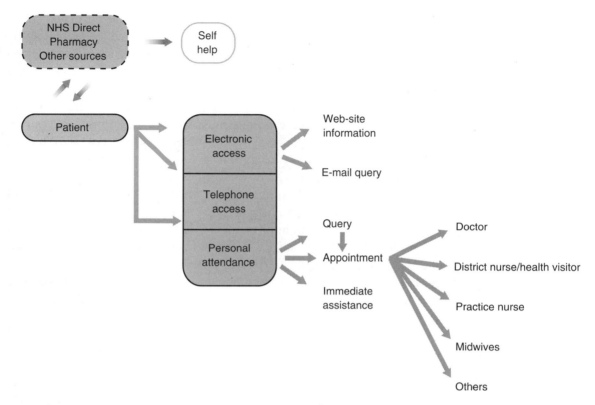

Figure 16.2 *The effect of the new NHS structure on patients.*

into independent Primary Care Trusts (PCTs). By April 2002, 302 had made this transition. PCG/Ts were saddled with heavy expectations. In obvious respects they represented an evolutionary advance – 'universalising the best of fundholding' – but the creation of budgets encompassing general medical services, prescribing, hospital and specialist care remained a major step forward. How have they fared?

Tracking progress   Establishing the organisation was a key early preoccupation and PCG/Ts made sound progress in their first 2 years. They have begun to translate priorities into clear local health strategies, targets and action plans. However, important challenges need to be addressed if PCTs are to realise their undoubted potential (Smith et al 2000, Wilkin et al 2001).

Not all PCT boards function in a corporate manner, and GPs sometimes dominate board meetings at the expense of contributions from nurses, social services and lay members! There remain significant concerns about the degree to which practices are effectively engaged in the work of PCTs, and about the relative lack of progress in involving lay stakeholders. Management budgets varied widely between PCTs, with clear consequences for their organisational development.

PCTs are getting to grips with their responsibilities for managing budgets, including the management of service level agreements and the development of incentive schemes, but many lack the necessary information and financial management capacity. A combination of unrealistic targets, a lack of resources and the inadequacy of existing systems is seriously impeding the ability of PCTs to generate the information needed to carry out their core functions.

Many PCTs have made considerable progress in developing minimum standards for practice services, agreeing plans for redistributing resources and making service improvements. Most have made a good start in establishing an infrastructure for clinical governance and initiating a range of activities involving practices and other staff. Much more remains to be done, however, in finding ways of tackling poor performance and dealing with 'outliers'. And in fact, many PCTs have struggled to support commissioning or health improvement. Although most PCTs have begun to develop closer links with social services departments, relationships with the wider local authority are limited at this stage. Boundary differences remain an obstacle to closer partnership working. Finally, the traditional clinical focus on the individual patient needs to be counterbalanced by a stronger focus on population health. Medical models of health and health care need to be supplemented by wider definitions of health and support for the interventions necessary to address the social determinants of ill health.

In summary, PCTs are developing as organisations at different speeds. They have made progress in developing and integrating primary and community care but their commissioning and health improvement functions as yet are limited. There is a danger that national policy imperatives, central directives and guidance will stifle the development of local policies addressing local needs.

After nearly a decade of rhetoric in support of the 'primary care-led NHS', there is little evidence of a shift in the balance of NHS expenditure (Gillam 2000). In absolute terms, it is the acute sector that continues to attract most new money. In many areas, PCG mergers give PCTs the aura and scale of the health authorities they replaced. Will PCTs have the critical mass they need to lever resources from hospitals into community-based services? Or will they fossilise as their bureaucracies burgeon rather than develop the agility needed for efficient commissioning? In the meantime, for many GPs they offer new opportunities to develop clinical and managerial skills.

Personal medical services – the quiet revolution

Although initially eclipsed by PCGs, Labour eventually extended the personal medical services (PMS) initiative. The PMS pilots proved unexpectedly popular after a slow start. By April 2002 nearly a quarter of all GPs were working under PMS. They are preferentially distributed at this stage in urban, more deprived areas, where the salaried option has been heavily taken up. Some of the financial risks of running a practice are reduced and, unsurprisingly, a reduction in the bureaucratic burdens of the job is welcome to many GPs. Salaried GPs appear to be happier with their income and hours of work than GMS GPs (National PMS Evaluation Team 2000).

It is hard to know how much service development can properly be attributed to PMS. First-wave pilots received an average of £62900 extra on entering PMS, but there is as yet little evidence that they are delivering improvements in patient care in comparison with GMS practices (Steiner 2001).

PMS provides entrepreneurs with some of the independence enjoyed by fundholders, and its success partly reflects its appeal to practices disaffected with the current reforms. Paradoxically, many practices see PMS as a way of defining their own priorities and insulating themselves from the intrusions of PCTs. Nevertheless, PMS provides crucial leverage for the PCTs that will in future hold their contracts. For the first time, PCTs hold truly integrated budgets with the ability to commission local primary care. Where all practices are contracted to their local PCT, the vision of a UK-style health maintenance organisation is already being realised.

> **L** In matters of party politics, and where personal choices of styles of practice are concerned, there are, for exam purposes, no 'right' or 'wrong' answers. All that will be expected of candidates is that they hold justifiable opinions based on sound evidence and core general practice values.

Addressing variations in quality

Variations in the quality of primary care, particularly in inner cities, have been a prominent concern of policy-makers since the inception of the NHS. The Conservative Government sought to import organisation-wide quality improvement strategies perceived as successful in manufacturing and service industries. The 1989 White Paper *Working for Patients* extolled the virtues of audit (Secretary of State for Health 1989). In some disciplines, 'the critical analysis of the quality of health care' was already established as best practice. What was new was an attempt to generalise audit activity. Over £500 million was spent on audit in the hospital and community sectors to mixed effect. The audit movement fell short of expectations in various ways (Spencer 1993). Audit topics reflected the priorities of doctors with little non-medical involvement. It proved difficult to routinise audit activity and involvement remained patchy. Clinical audit did not engage the traditionally 'hard to reach'. Participation in audit was voluntary and not a contractual obligation upon GPs.

The invention of clinical governance by the Labour Government heralded the latest of many attempts in the NHS to exercise greater managerial control over clinical activities. Governmental concerns over professional self-regulation were heightened in the wake of events at the Bristol Royal Infirmary and were about to be raised still more dramatically.

Clinical governance has been defined as a system through which NHS organisations are accountable for continuously improving the quality of

Box 16.1
The scope of clinical governance in primary care

■ Clear lines of responsibility and accountability for the overall quality of clinical care
■ A comprehensive programme of quality improvement activities:
  (a) evidence-based practice
  (b) National Service Frameworks/NICE
  (c) workforce planning and development
  (d) continuing professional development
  (e) safeguarding patient confidentiality
  (f) clinical audit and outcomes
  (g) quality assurance
  (h) research and development
■ Risk management
■ Identification and remedy of poor performance

their services and safeguarding high standards of care by creating an environment in which clinical excellence will flourish (NHS Executive 1998). It draws together elements of quality assurance that are often poorly coordinated. The corporate nature of this new responsibility requires, in the overused phrase, major 'cultural change'. For PCTs, this implies sharing intelligence about quality across professional and practice boundaries, and health professionals seeing themselves as collectively accountable for the clinical and cost effectiveness of their colleagues' work. Box 16.1 illustrates the scope of clinical governance in primary care.

Clinical governance presents particular challenges for PCTs. In setting their own clinical governance priorities they will have to reconcile national 'givens' with local concerns if the priorities they identify are to be 'owned' by their constituents. They need to link forward planning and implementation of clinical governance with primary care investment and the implementation of their local health improvement programme (HImP). Clinical governance implies a new understanding about the nature of professional accountability. Is there any evidence of progress where previous attempts to improve quality of care have failed?

Progress on clinical governance

There are wide differences between the amount that PCGs planned to spend on clinical governance. This in turn ensured variable levels of local support in the form of new staff (Wilkin et al 2001). Many clinical governance leads are scrambling up steep learning curves and only now are beginning to understand the complexity of their jobs (Hayward et al 1999). In the majority of PCTs, practices have appointed their own clinical governance lead. However, levels of support from other agencies, such as public health departments, academic bodies or education networks vary considerably (Hayward et al 1999). Links with clinical governance structures in the acute sector are developing slowly.

One enduring challenge is the search for a package of performance indicators to help identify substandard performance. The easily measurable is rarely useful. Technical obstacles, such as the difficulties of controlling for case-mix, are not easily resolved. Most indicators are influenced by factors outside the control of health systems. Evidence-based measures of process will perhaps continue to be more useful than measures of outcome.

The management of poor performance presents PCTs with a major challenge. Complaints, colleagues' expressed concerns and financial audit visits by the health authority were the traditional means of detection. The consultation paper *Supporting Doctors, Protecting Patients* (NHS Executive 1999a) proposed compulsory annual audit and appraisal for all doctors, with assessment and support centres for failing doctors, but it is not yet clear how these will operate.

The emphasis has been on setting the right cultural tone as much as on concrete achievements. In the wake of the Shipman verdict, this has not been easy. PCTs are trying to adopt a non-threatening, facilitative and developmental approach to clinical governance while setting up new local monitoring mechanisms (Wye et al 2000). The threats to both independent contractor status and professional self-regulation have increased doctors' feelings of beleaguerment. They are unconvinced by the rhetoric of a 'no blame' culture.

The access card

The Labour administration was no less concerned than its predecessors to ensure timely access to care. The first National Patients Survey confirmed that difficulties booking appointments and waiting times for routine or emergency care were prominent public concerns (NHS Executive 1999b). Fair access formed one dimension of a new performance assessment framework but, at first sight, the raft of policy initiatives designed to improve access to primary care appeared populist and reflexive. NHS Direct, the nurse-led telephone helpline, was to provide 'easier and faster advice and information for people about health, illness and the NHS so that they are better able to care for themselves and their families'. More specific objectives for NHS Direct included the encouragement of self-care at home and reducing unnecessary use of other NHS services, that is, management of demand (Rosen & Florin 1999).

GPs were sceptical of claims that NHS Direct would reduce their workloads. They were quick to seize on 'evidence' to rationalise the extension of the service country-wide. The final report confirmed that the new service has had little impact on other emergency services (Munro et al 2000).

Already sensitive to threats to their professional monopoly over first contact care, the medical profession was therefore doubly wary of the introduction of walk-in centres. These were a specific response to the apparent success of instant access primary care facilities established by the private sector, notably on railway stations serving time-pressed commuters. Anything Medicentres could provide, the NHS could provide better. More serious concerns revolved around the experience of walk-in centres in other countries, notably Canada (Jones 2000). Multiple access points with poorly coordinated record keeping could result in fragmented care. Most of the first 36 were to be nurse-led. Walk-in centres were there-fore easily conflated with other threats to the future of independent contractor status.

In summary, these innovations nicely crystallised the differences in priority different players attach to access. Their apparent popularity with patients contrasted with their reluctant acceptance by health professionals, but concerns over their cost effectiveness remain.

New labour, new crises ... new Plan

Labour's was a 10-year project and the development of effective PCTs was always going to take more time than the 5-year electoral cycle allowed. Similarly, the implementation of clinical governance was never going to keep health scandals from the national news. *The NHS Plan* was published to maintain the momentum in the modernisation of the NHS (NHS Executive 2000). Public failures, particularly those of the medical profession, armed the Government to challenge entrenched medical interests and strengthened the case for reform.

The NHS Plan was supposed to represent a 'new deal' between the Government and the health sector (Box 16.2). In return for substantial new funding, the Government sought to challenge some of the long-established foundations of the NHS and, in particular, to revisit the settlement between organised medicine and the State. Alternative methods of funding health care (private insurance, co-payments, social insurance) were, however, explicitly rejected. What does all this presage for general practice?

An expansion in hospital beds and consultant numbers, with consequent reductions in waiting times, if realised, should ease the burden of

Box 16.2
The NHS Plan – key points

- 500 one-stop health centres by 2004
- 3000 surgeries upgraded by 2004
- 2000 more GPs and 450 more registrars by 2004
- NHS Lift, a new private–public partnership, to develop premises
- 1000 specialist GPs
- Consultants delivering 4 million outpatient appointments in primary care
- 2100 extra acute and general hospital beds
- 5000 extra intermediate care beds
- Outpatient appointments to drop from 6 to 3 months
- Patients given copies of clinicians' letters
- Single-handed GPs to sign up to 'new contractual quality standards'
- Annual appraisals from 2002
- Mandatory audit from 2002 to support revalidation
- The GMC to be part of new umbrella organisation of regulatory bodies
- Assessment centres to oversee doctors' performance from 2001

containment in primary care. At present, the expansion of GP numbers is less impressive, representing only a modest increase in long-term trends. Even allowing for investment in other community-based services, GPs will not easily be able to improve access to their services or extend consultation lengths.

Increasingly, patients who currently go to hospital will be able to have tests and treatment in one of 500 new primary care centres. Consultants who previously worked only in hospitals will be seeing outpatients in these settings and 'GPs with special interests' will be taking referrals from their colleagues in fields such as ophthalmology, orthopaedics and dermatology. The model for these is untested.

NHS Direct opens up new approaches to demand management. The vision is of a single phone call to the one-stop gateway to all out-of-hours health care. Many primary care providers will be nurse-led and ostensibly more cost-efficient. The same substitution of less expensive human resources is reflected in new extended roles for pharmacists. Nurses are being equipped to take on hitherto medical tasks in line with their North American counterparts. Similarly, GP subspecialists will take on work previously undertaken by hospital consultants.

Progress on partnership building at the level of the PCT is as yet patchy. The jury is out on whether these organisations can really work effectively to tackle the determinants of health inequalities. Although they are only slowly developing their commissioning functions, PCTs provide a vehicle for the increasing integration of health and social care. The proposed Care Trusts, bringing together health and social services funds, are unlikely to overcome all the long-standing barriers to joint working at this interface but they remain a logical progression.

The quid pro quo – and a new contract

If *The NHS Plan* signals a major investment in new staff and facilities, the Government clearly expects more than just 'principled motivation' in return. The early emphasis by the Labour Government on increased regulation of professionals is considerably strengthened under the Plan. The most significant change to the ways GPs work has been the elaboration of a new contractual framework building on the stipulations for improved outcomes that are supposed to be inherent in the PMS approach. In future, GP pay will be linked more closely to workload and quality of care.

The Labour Government has been criticised for its centralising tendencies at the expense of local experimentation. Although couched in a vocabulary suggesting local discretion, *The NHS Plan* tightens central control (Lewis & Gillam 2001). New accountability structures are being created. The Modernisation Agency and other task-forces are overseeing implementation and a new super-regulator, the Commission for Healthcare Audit and Inspection (CHAI), is being created. Whatever the Government's intentions, some clinicians and managers fear they will be operating within an environment that is increasingly dominated by predetermined clinical frameworks and an enhanced performance management framework.

However, subject to satisfactory performance, NHS bodies are promised considerable freedom from central supervision and interference ('earned autonomy'). Ironically, the latest pronouncements giving 'foundation trusts' new freedoms to use private finance presage something like the Conservatives' internal market.

Conclusions

In 1997 the out-going Conservative Government presented the incoming Labour administration with many of the tools it has wielded in its quest for modernisation. The internal market has been adapted in gradualist fashion within a framework of mandatory collective funding. In other respects, the Labour Government has proved unexpectedly radical. Least clearly foreseen was the series of initiatives designed to change the nature of first contact and to free up access to health care.

Demographic and other pressures on the primary care workforce carry their own imperatives. Persisting nurse shortages and the retirement of a cadre of overseas-trained GPs serving inner city populations determine the need for new networks of provision. Both within and out of hours, it seems likely that a plurality of nurse-led providers will form the first point of contact.

The collectivisation of primary care under Labour marks a move towards managed care under UK-style health maintenance organisations. The PMS initiative heralded the end of a single national contract and changes the nature of independent contractor status. Much generalist care will be provided not by individual practitioners but from inter-professional units under local contracts. As today's surgeries increasingly become the service outlets for larger primary care organisations, many 'corner shops' will disappear.

A key strength of UK general practice has been its comprehensive financing system. There are risks in unravelling the GPs' national contract – but potential gains too. Top-down governance is acknowledged as having failed to provide the innovation or responsiveness to deliver sustained improvement in patient care. The new contract seeks more effectively to link pay to workload and to reward quality. It should encourage local entrepreneurs.

L 'Quality' is a constantly recurring concept in debate about models of healthcare delivery, particularly where it can be linked to issues of appraisal and remuneration. What do you personally mean by 'high-quality practice', and how could you demonstrate to an evaluator that you provide it?

In future, GPs will no longer be the only hub around which primary care revolves, but they need not fear 'modernisation'. Long after today's new structures have disappeared, people will be seeking the personal care that tomorrow's general practice should strive to provide. Returning to a theme of the opening paragraphs, it has become a cliché in the health service to state that the one certainty facing health professionals is constant change. Following the Wanless report, the Labour Government looks set to commit major new investment to the health service in the coming years, thereby fulfilling its pledge to raise funding levels to European averages (Wanless 2002). The number of GPs looks set to expand along with many new opportunities to diversify the role. For new entrants to general practice, old certainties may be changing but you have made an exciting choice.

> **L** While the MRCGP is a UK-based exam, it is not above asking about other models of primary care, such as those found in European, North American and Antipodean countries, particularly where we might have lessons to learn from them.

Summary

- Containing costs, increasing efficiency, addressing variations in clinical quality, increasing professional accountability and improving access and responsiveness have been government priorities for the NHS since the 1980s.

- 'Fundholding' was introduced in 1990 by the Conservative Government in an attempt to provide an 'internal market' in health care. It failed to deliver the expected efficiency gains.

- In 1997, the Labour Government introduced primary care groups to replace fundholding and moved to replace the internal market with unified budgets and a duty of partnership between the different elements within the NHS (general practice, hospital and community health services).

- On behalf of their local populations, primary care groups had three main functions: to improve health and address inequalities, to develop primary and community health services, and to commission a range of community and hospital services. Over time, all primary care groups evolved into independent primary care trusts.

- Personal medical services (PMS) reduces some of the financial risks of running a practice and is proving very popular – especially in more deprived urban areas where the salaried option has been heavily taken up.

- Clinical governance is now the system by which variations in quality of health provision are being eradicated. Following high-profile cases, such as that of Harold Shipman, clinical governance has assumed an even greater prominence than it originally had in the area of professional self-regulation.

■ *The NHS Plan* was published in 2000. In return for substantial new Government funding, the Plan challenged some long-established NHS traditions. In particular, the regulation of health professionals has been strengthened and new accountability structures have been introduced. There has also been a series of initiatives designed to change the nature of first contact and to free up access to health care.

■ The new GP contract seeks to link GP pay to workload, and to reward quality. The number of GPs is gradually expanding and there are many new opportunities to diversify the GP role.

References

Audit Commission 1996 What the doctor ordered: a study of GP fundholding in England and Wales. HMSO, London

Department of Health 1997a The NHS (Primary Care) Act 1997. HMSO, London

Department of Health 1997b The new NHS: modern, dependable. HMSO, London

Department of Health 1998 The new NHS: modern and dependable. Primary care groups: delivering the agenda (HSC 1998/288). Department of Health, Leeds

Gillam S 2000 Homeward bound? Just how far have we come in re-directing resources to primary care? Health Management November:14–15

Hayward J, Rosen R, Dewar S 1999 Thin on the ground. Health Services Journal 26 August:6–27

Jones M 2000 Walk-in primary care centres: lessons from Canada. British Medical Journal 321: 928–931

Le Grand J, Mays N, Mulligan J (eds) 1998 Learning from the NHS internal market. A review of the evidence. King's Fund, London

Lewis R, Gillam S (eds) 1999 Transforming primary care. Personal medical services in the new NHS. King's Fund, London

Lewis R, Gillam S 2001 The NHS Plan – further reform of the British health service. International Journal of Health Services 31:111–118

Mays N, Goodwin N, Killoran A, Malbon G on behalf of the Total Purchasing National Evaluation Team 1999 Total purchasing: a step towards primary care groups. King's Fund, London

Munro J, Nicholl J, O'Cathain A, Knowles E 2000 Evaluation of NHS Direct first wave sites. Second interim report to the Department of Health.

Medical Care Research Unit, University of Sheffield, Sheffield

National PMS Evaluation Team 2000 National evaluation of first wave NHS personal medical services pilots: integrated interim report from four research projects. National Primary Care Research and Development Centre, Manchester

NHS Executive 1994 Developing NHS purchasing and GP fundholding: towards a primary care-led NHS (EL(94)79). HMSO, London

NHS Executive 1998 A first class service: quality in the new NHS. Department of Health, London

NHS Executive 1999a Supporting doctors, protecting patients. HMSO, London

NHS Executive 1999b The national surveys of NHS patients. General practice 1998. Department of Health, London

NHS Executive 2000 The NHS Plan. A plan for investment. A plan for reform (CM 4818-I). HMSO, London

Rosen R, Florin D 1999 Evaluating NHS Direct. British Medical Journal 319:5–6

Secretaries of State for Health in England, Wales and Scotland 1996 Choice and opportunity. Primary care: the future. HMSO, London

Secretary of State for Health 1989 Working for patients (CM 555.78). HMSO, London

Smith J, Regen E, Goodwin N et al 2000 Getting into their stride. Interim report of a national evaluation of primary care groups. University of Birmingham, Health Services Management Centre, Birmingham

Spencer J 1993 Audit in general practice: where do we go from here? Quality in Health Care 2:183–188

Steiner A (ed) 2001 Does PMS improve quality of care? Final report from the quality of care project, national evaluation of PMS. NPCRDC/University of Southampton, Southampton

Wanless D 2002 Securing our future health: taking a long term view. HM Treasury, London

Wilkin D, Gillam S, Coleman A (eds) 2001 The national tracker survey of primary care groups and trusts: modernizing the NHS, 2000/2001. National Primary Care Research and Development Centre/King's Fund, London

Wye L, Rosen R, Dewar S 2000 Clinical governance in primary care. A review of baseline assessments. King's Fund, London

17

How does a practice work? The role of a practice manager

Dee Stenning, Surinder Singh

L   MRCGP examiners are often disappointed in the level of registrars' knowledge of practice management and finance. Some candidates appear reluctant to accept that general practice functions as a 'small business', to which the principles of good management can and should be applied.

At the time the National Health Service began in 1948 the tradition was for general practitioners to work alone, often from one or two rooms in their home. In such times there was no 'manager' and the only support might be from the doctor's spouse or one receptionist. As services became more organised in the years that followed, groups of two and three doctors started to form partnerships and administrative needs emerged in terms of organising rooms, allocating jobs, and face-to-face personnel skills. More staff were taken on, often neighbours or friends of the GP recruited more for their good nature than any specific skills or experience. There were few, if any, formal systems for anything.

Today, GPs typically work in a group practice where three or more partners work together in various full- and part-time or job-share combinations. They might well employ one or more non-principals to share the medical workload. They will almost certainly work with a practice nurse and a primary care team, using computer technology to manage clinical information, prescribing and quality monitoring systems for their patients.

Many of the changes highlighted above took off after the 1966 General Practice Charter (Fry 1993), when practices that were often struggling financially were encouraged to use partly funded healthcare staff to improve overall care. This resulted in much greater use of employed staff in the surgery.

The late 1970s and early 1980s saw the merging of smaller practices and the availability of cost-rent funding for improvements in premises. Practice nursing, previously a fairly low-status activity, gradually increased in prominence and was further strengthened through the 1990 GP Contract, with its emphasis on health promotion activity. The gradual introduction of computerised clinical systems was encouraged and partially financed by health authorities as information technology advanced during the 1980s and 1990s. All of this led to a need for greater emphasis on 'management' within the practice.

Initially, GPs took on most of the management functions themselves, with some delegation to receptionists and nurses. The widespread employment of managers in general practice is therefore a relatively new phenomenon, which really only took off after the 1990 GP Contract, especially in those practices that took on fundholding under the last Conservative Government. More recently, new ways of providing primary care, for example Personal Medical Services (PMS) pilot schemes, have emerged. These approaches to healthcare provision, run by GPs, nurses and practice managers, aim to enable care to be targeted and more focused on local needs, rather than along traditional General Medical Services (GMS) lines (see Chapter 16).

The formation of PMS pilots, which enable practices and others to provide services in new and innovative ways, means that all the members of the primary healthcare team will need to take responsibility and have an active part in managing resources, not only for primary care but for secondary care also. Suddenly, new skills are required of practice managers, shifting from the role of receptionist and administrator to that of business or general manager. Managers and administrative staff have to be proactive in their continuing development and learning needs if they are to ensure that they have a job in the future.

As a registrar, you will by definition work in a training practice. Such practices tend to be large and are likely to employ a manager. With all the new aspects of clinical work you have to deal with you might feel that you can leave the management to the managers. Remember, however, that not all practices you work in subsequently will employ a manager. In those that do not, all the managerial functions described in this chapter must still be fulfilled and, ultimately, the partners in any practice are responsible for its smooth running.

What is the role of today's practice manager?

A practice manager is responsible for a diverse range of functions (Box 17.1).

The skills needed to manage a practice effectively are numerous. As well as knowledge and understanding of the principles of business management, good communication skills are essential as much of the work involves dealing with people, be they the doctors, other members of the primary healthcare team, patients, carers and the numerous outside services with whom the practice deals. It is also essential to have an assertive and confident manner to control difficult situations that might arise. Keeping calm and having a sense of humour can help in such circumstances.

> **L** Questions often appear in the written paper for which a grasp of some of the formal principles of business management would be helpful. Airport departure lounge bookstores are full of books on this topic, and the works of Belbin (1996), e.g. *Why Teams Fail*, can be recommended.

The following is a brief summary of some of the essential areas of practice management.

Box 17.1
A summary of a practice manager's role

■ Financial management:
  – PAYE
  – pensions
  – national insurance
■ Strategic development of practice:
  – clinical governance
  – risk management
■ Patient welfare
■ Human resource management:
  – practice staff
■ Information management and technology
■ Management of facilities (including building)

Financial management

PAYE

- Paying staff on a monthly basis, including Statutory Sick Pay and Statutory Maternity Pay. Paying Tax and National Insurance to the Inland Revenue, operating NHS Pension scheme requirements.
- Completing P14s at end of tax year on all employees.
- Sending P45s, P46s and P15s to tax office for new employees.
- Completing P45s for employees leaving.
- Use of deduction working sheets and wages book or appropriate computer system.

> **L** It is worth talking at length with your practice manager and your trainer about the practice accounts, and how to interpret information supplied by the practice's accountant. Apart from its relevance when you come to study the balance sheet of a practice you are considering joining, there is no reason why financial information should not be presented as material for analysis in the MRCGP written paper.

Banking

- Paying bills on a weekly/monthly basis and receiving bank cheques weekly.

Cash books and accounting

- Establishing and keeping accurate, timely and balanced accounting systems through cash books and computerised systems.
- Reconciling monthly bank statements to cash books.
- Acting as first point of contact for bank, accountants, auditors and partners.
- Ensuring all documentation is in place for the preparation of annual accounts with the practice auditors.
- Preparing cash-flow forecasts.
- Operating the devolved staff budget in liaison with GPs and being responsible for submission and reimbursement of claims.
- Exploring ways of increasing income (e.g. targets, items of service work and reporting areas of underperformance to the partners).
- Monitoring insurance policies and ensuring payments are up-to-date.

Petty cash books

- Monitoring and controlling petty cash.
- Ensuring accountability for petty cash is clear.

Practice strategic development, clinical governance and risk management

This is a vital area for the whole practice, not just the practice manager. Certainly the vogue for clinical governance, patient safety and procedures to ensure the highest quality care means that the practice manager will be involved to some degree. A common approach is that each practice appoints a clinical governance 'lead' – who might be the practice manager but does not have to be. Other practices take a more democratic approach and ensure that all members of the practice take a lead in their own areas of interest (see Chapter 8 for more on clinical governance). Thus, a practice manager's role in this area might include:

- Coordinating the production of practice development plans and reports.
- Coordinating clinical audit processes as directed by the clinical governance lead and coordination of organisational audit with the partners, reviewing and disseminating the results.
- Ensuring compliance with local arrangements and systems for delivering evidence-based practice, generating data as required. This might involve being the central coordinator for all complaints, including those that involve clinical staff (see also Chapter 11).
- Chairing primary healthcare team meetings where appropriate and implementing action plans.
- Formulating up-to-date practice leaflets.

The practice leaflet   It was a requirement introduced in the 1990 GP contract that a practice leaflet is produced and made available to patients. This document should include basic information about the practice including:

- personal and professional details of the doctors
- availability of doctors and nurses and any designated clinics
- use of the appointment system and methods of obtaining home visits
- out-of-hours arrangements
- information regarding clinics and availability of maternity medical services.

At present, most people choose their doctor by such criteria as location. Clearly, as a patient, it is important to find a doctor you can trust and who provides the services you need. A well-prepared practice leaflet should enable an informed choice to be made. In addition, it can also help long-standing patients of the practice to find out about services that are provided within the practice. It does, however, raise a number of interesting points. For example:

- Are doctors allowed to advertise their services? It is illegal at present for doctors to say that they are the best GPs in the country and that other doctors down the road should never have been allowed to set up in practice. It is allowable to say that you provide a first-class quality service.
- Where can you put your practice leaflet? Certainly it can be left on the practice premises. It is also permissible to leave copies in the local library, the community clinic, or with the estate agent in the high street.
- How do you pay for your leaflet? Producing a publication of any sort uses resources, principally time and money. Consequently, it seems logical to try and reduce those costs by obtaining some form of sponsorship, for example from local businesses. Of course, obvious conflicts can occur if this funding is from a drug company or even a local chemist.

Thus the production of a practice leaflet can bring its own problems. Nevertheless, it also brings an opportunity to ensure that the local population is aware of the services you provide, and can offer an intriguing insight into the practice and the people who work in it.

The annual report　A report must be provided annually to the primary care organisation (PCO) by the doctor, relating to the provision by him or her of personal medical services. This should contain the following:

- staff numbers and duties
- details of practice premises
- referral of patients to specialists
- the doctor's other commitments as medical practitioner
- arrangements for patients' comments on the provision of general medical services
- use of formularies and repeat prescriptions.

A practice annual report requires the collection of information by the practice and is a statutory obligation of the GP contract. This is a chance to look at and perhaps reflect on what you are doing, how you are doing it and the costs therein – not just monetary. Potentially, it is a management tool for yourself and the practice, and tells you a lot about the practice. It depends on the accurate collection of information. This requires disease registers, an accurate count of referrals and procedures carried out in the practice. In addition, it requires use of time and resources to compile, time that could be spent otherwise, for example, in seeing patients.

Information management and technology　Information technology (IT) (see also Chapter 18) should help make the work of the practice more efficient and enhance patient care. This will only happen if systems are properly managed and used. Data of all sorts can be stored and organised on modern clinical computer systems, which can also provide a powerful form of communication within the practice and with outside agencies such as the PCT, Health Authority and local hospitals. In many practices the smooth running and the team's ability to use the full potential of information technology depends on the interests and knowledge of the practice manager.

The practice manager's specific tasks in this area are:

- Ensuring the maintenance of computer management and systems – whatever the system.
- Using the computer system to search and audit facilities.
- Analysing and reconciling the output of GP links data, ensuring the production of quarterly reports.
- Undertaking research, where appropriate, and make recommendations and establish new 'care' systems as required.
- Negotiating of servicing and maintenance of computer hardware.
- Taking the lead on IT development and overseeing all systems for data security and protection, including back-up facilities.

Patient welfare

This role is crucial to and for the practice. It is this area that ensures that the needs of patients are being addressed, and hopefully met. Thus how to convey information to patients, people and families is the central role here:

- Taking responsibility for the production of practice information such as practice leaflets, newsletters, appointment cards.
- Producing and reviewing marketing plans for the practice to market services.
- Planning and reviewing clinics in response to patient need and profile of the practice.
- Producing and updating practice complaint procedures in collaboration with the partners.
- Dealing with patient queries and complaints (see also Human resource management below).
- Encouraging and maintaining patients' participation in the practice, including requests for feedback and production of evaluation tools.
- Liaising with clinical and community organisations.

Management of building facilities

- Taking responsibility for devising and maintaining systems for purchasing supplies and equipment.
- Organising maintenance schedules, recommending purchase of new pieces of equipment, undertaking feasibility studies.
- Liaising with other parts of the building and with maintenance and cleaning services (e.g. if in a health centre, ensuring that all parts of the building used by the practice are well maintained and cleaned).
- Ensuring consulting rooms are fully equipped at all times.
- Ensuring the surgery premises are kept safe, tidy, pleasant and welcoming. Ensuring that security is tested and reviewed regularly.
- Ensuring that the practice complies with the Health and Safety legislation and alerting all staff to these policies and procedures.
- Assisting the partners in the development of the premises, including overseeing the financial control and project management for equipment or premises upgrades.

Human resource management

The major task under this category is the 'hiring and firing of staff'. This means that recruiting, being part of the interviews, selecting and inducting new staff are all involved in this process. Other related tasks include:

- Drawing up criteria for the vacancy, producing or revising job descriptions, advertising vacancies, short-listing, obtaining references and clearances, interviewing, employment and issuing contracts and policies.
- Coordinating arrangements for partnership change, including the recruitment and selection process for appointing new partners.

- Producing and overseeing training and induction programmes for all staff.
- Ensuring staff appraisals take place for all staff and carrying out one-to-one appraisal reviews with administrative and reception staff.
- Keeping up-to-date with employment legislation, making necessary changes and drawing these to the attention of all staff.
- Ensuring staff are working well and as a team and exploring areas of underperformance, including the implementation of disciplinary procedures.
- Developing and maintaining policies and procedures for the practice including:
  - managing the staff budget and being involved in bidding for staff budgets
  - organising and attending staff meetings, including establishing agendas, ensuring minutes are taken and distributed, reviewing actions.
- Identifying staff training needs and coordinating individual and practice training sessions.
- Establishing and monitoring staff rotas and monitoring staff holidays and absences.

Case illustration

It is often thought that how a practice deals with a complaint is a fair indicator of how it deals with patients and people in general. Imagine that, in your practice, an experienced partner has a complaint lodged against him and the patient is threatening to 'take him to the General Medical Council'. There is one problem – the difficult consultation took place 18 months ago and the partner is thinking about dismissing it because it is 'out of time'.

What is the practice manager's role in dealing fairly with this complaint and who should be supporting the partner in dealing with it (see also Chapter 11)?

Practice staff

General information

The number of staff employed by GPs doubled between 1984 and 1994. At the same time, reception, secretarial and clerical staff accounted for two-thirds of staff and practice managers for 12% (NHS Executive 1996). The shift away from secondary care emphasises the importance placed on primary care in delivering services and explains why there has been an increase in practice staff. The increased emphasis on quality, performance, efficiency, effectiveness and value for money reflects changes that have occurred over the last 10 years. There is an increased emphasis on management, leadership and teamwork and there have been significant changes in the balance of skills within the professional groups, resulting in generic workers, multiskilled professionals and generic support staff. Other changes in the twenty-first century might mean that there will be fewer managers. The advent of primary care organisations

(PCOs) means that Trusts and GPs will be working more closely together and there will be pressure to reduce management costs. This will affect the numbers of managers needed, and means a tightening in this labour market. However, competencies and skills will become increasingly important so continuous training for all those involved is vital. Both Cottam et al (1994) and Fitzgerald (1990) have identified the need for managers within health care to develop multifunctional skills. If the proposals outlined in *The New NHS: Modern and Dependable* (NHS Executive 1998) are to be fulfilled, managers must have the support and the opportunity to develop the necessary skills.

Practice staff

Could you manage without your receptionist? Could you do the job as well as he or she does? Why are most receptionists women (this is supposed to be an age of equality)? Could you face dealing with irate members of the public who complain that they can't see their doctor for days? Who would take this sort of poorly paid job and tolerate the difficulties that it may bring with it?

There must be advantages to the job or GPs wouldn't be able to get any staff at all! So why do people work as receptionists? What are they expected to do? Are they disposable lackeys or indispensable members of a team? Do they act to protect the doctor from 'difficult' patients or enable worried and ill people to get access to a medical service?

From the GP's viewpoint, reception staff are needed to help them provide a service to their patients, for example by running administrative systems and managing the process of access to care and communication with outside agencies. It is clear that different staff are needed for different tasks, although there might be considerable overlap between which person carries out which task. A brief list of staff required may be as follows:

- receptionist
- telephonist
- filing clerk
- secretary
- computer operator
- practice nurses
- practice manager.

The advent of the practice administrator or practice manager has further aided GPs in delegation of responsibilities. A competent practice manager will be able to relieve GPs of much of the burden of administrative duties by looking after staff salaries, maintenance of buildings, ordering of drugs and equipment and various other tasks. Furthermore, a practice manager will be able to help with development of practice activities, whether this is expansion as a business or of premises, introduction of new equipment, employing new staff or expanding the range of medical services offered. For the practice manager to do this, though, he or she must necessarily have access to a lot of information on how the practice is run, the state of the finances, the plans for the partners – in other words the strategic position of the partners. This position can consequently be a difficult one.

For example, partners may be reluctant to provide what is regarded as sensitive information about future plans for practice development or partners' income, or be reluctant to involve the practice manager where there is a partnership dispute. Without trust and mutual understanding it will be almost impossible for the practice manager to perform the job. Furthermore, if the practice manager has responsibility for hiring and firing staff, then he or she may also come into contact with the other employees in the practice and, concomitantly, be seen as a blunt tool of 'the management'. In these circumstances it is vital that he or she has the support and confidence of the partners; if decisions taken are then impeded or reversed by the partners, the practice manager's position will be severely undermined.

Although the practice manager will be able to settle many of the problems and disputes that arise, it is important that the staff feel they can have access to the partners to reflect back on changes that might have occurred in the practice, the way the practice is running, to be able to provide ideas and suggestions and to air grievances, if appropriate. It would seem sensible, then, for the partners to keep in touch with the feelings and views of their staff, either on an individual, informal basis or by regular practice meetings. The relationship between staff and doctors is an important one and the happiness or otherwise of the practice is likely to be reflected in the approach to patients and their needs.

Morale Good staff morale is likely to improve service to the patients, enthusiasm towards attaining targets, and so on. A review of individual and overall performance should allow areas of competence and excellence to be recognised and areas of weakness to be discussed. If mistakes are continually picked up on, and competence and achievement pass unrecognised, morale is likely to be low and staff turnover high. Recognition can be verbal or written in terms of praise; with the new targets in practice it might be relevant to consider bonuses for performance as both a reward and an incentive, in addition to the traditional party or Christmas gifts.

Managers need to be able to deal with changes in an efficient and effective manner. To ensure that the services we provide are safe, we need to have a culture that is open and is a 'no blame' culture. A competent practice manager will be able to relieve GPs of much of the burden of administrative duties, the skills, knowledge and experience needed to do this effectively are listed below:

- a high degree of specialised knowledge and experience
- proven leadership skills

- good communication skills
- sound financial knowledge
- decision-making abilities
- ability to delegate and motivate
- ability to manage change effectively
- knowledge of employment law
- understanding of critical analysis and evaluation
- training skills
- good time management and able to establish priorities
- knowledge of Health and Safety at Work Act, Terms of Service and GP Contract
- commitment to working in a primary healthcare team.

What are the attributes for the job?

Clearly, the above points are a useful start in formulating an overall person specification for the role of practice manager. As we have said, it helps to be confident and calm to manage the many task involved in as effective and appropriate a way as possible.

One important area often not discussed is support. Networking amongst practice managers, sharing best practice and working with other managers in training and education helps create a cooperative approach to problems in a locality (Harrison & Redpath 1998). Innovation comes about when such a supportive environment has been created. Other sources of support include traditional methods (reading articles and books) and using the worldwide web. For an example of a website designed to 'act as a resource and provider of frameworks, advice and information', go to www.primeline.org.uk (Primeline 2001).

Conclusions

Practice managers play a pivotal role in the organisation of the delivery of health care to patients. Their roles and responsibilities in practice have changed during the last decade and are likely to undergo further changes in the future. Managers not only have to keep up-to-date with issues affecting their management in primary care, but also extend their knowledge, skills and understanding to meet the new requirements of working in partnership with patients and external agencies. The changes in the workings of community organisations (PCGs and PCTs) is just one example of this (Gillam 1999) (see also Chapter 16).

In a time of potential information overload, practice managers play the role of central communicator within the practice and often act as its voice, internally and externally, and speak for patients. The manager will sift and prioritise information and ensure that essential facts reach those who need them in a timely manner.

The practice needs to be managed in a cost-effective manner to ensure its profitability and the principals' incomes. Services need to be of a high quality and should also be responsive to the needs of patients.

This can only be achieved with the contribution of a well-motivated team, where individuals feel valued and are enthusiastic in delivering optimum care. The 'management' of this team is one of the keys to a successful practice. The ability of the practice manager to respond to the challenge of change and to be proactive will ensure that he or she is prepared for the future.

Training and education affects the development of the practice and this area should continue to be an integral part of planning and form part of the culture. The practice manager has a major part to play in ensuring that he or she is familiar with the structure and objectives of the training programme.

Induction is an important part of any staff member's training and assists anyone joining the practice in settling into the new environment and understanding the culture and mindset of the practice. The practice manager needs to ensure that all staff who join the practice – and this includes GP registrars, new partners and salaried GPs – should undergo an induction programme. Having a checklist that details what is going to happen over a certain period of time is useful not only for the practice but also for the new employee or doctor.

The manager's role includes strategic planning for the practice and the preparation, along with the rest of the management team, of a practice business plan, which should set out the aims and objectives of the practice for the next 2 or 3 years. Many do not think it practical to plan more than 3 years ahead, although medium-term planning, for example around new premises, might need to be 'factored in' as the practice grows.

Managers are also responsible for ensuring that the practice complies with current legislation, and this includes such areas as data protection, computer security, and health and safety. This type of structural responsibility also pertains to other areas, such as overseeing patient confidentiality, and the practice manager is central to this as well.

Team-building, that is, ensuring the practice runs smoothly and that staff are all pulling in the same direction and that there is a general shared understanding of the practice aims and objectives, is a major responsibility of the practice manager.

There must be staff involvement in decision making, and consultation to ensure that any changes introduced are accepted and understood by all. If there is no ownership, changing working practice or introducing new services will be difficult. The manager's role in ensuring this happens is crucial to the smooth running of the practice.

It is perhaps glib to state that a modern practice manager has a multi-faceted role within the practice. As this chapter illustrates, the secret to the manager's role is ensuring that structures, people and systems are managed in such a way that output is optimal, stress levels are minimised and people are happy (Fig. 17.1).

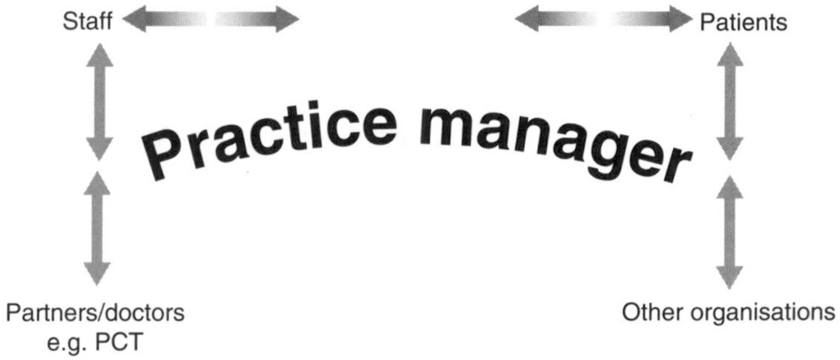

Figure 17.1
The position of the modern practice manager.

Summary

- The management of the practice is a task – or various tasks – that have to be fulfilled to ensure patient safety, smooth working, sound financial systems and a happy workforce. In this chapter, the approach has been to use a dedicated practice manager; however, this is only one way of ensuring effective practice management.

- Effective practice management means that a more formal management approach is utilised, for example in areas such as financial and business planning, employment of staff, information technology and, importantly, the overall strategy of the practice in the context of patient care.

L Should the management structure of a practice be fundamentally hierarchical? And if so, who is at the top and where should a practice manager come in the hierarchy? Or should it be more egalitarian? If so, should the manager be an employee of the practice or take a share of the profits, like the partners do?

References

Belbin RM 1996 Why teams fail. Butterworth-Heinemann, Oxford

Cottam D, Higgins J, Mahon A et al 1994 How to be top. Health Service Journal 104(5407):26–28

Fitzgerald L 1990 Management development in the NHS: crossing professional boundaries. Public Money and Management 10(1):31–35

Fry J 1993 The health team. General practice: the facts. Radcliffe Medical Press, Abingdon, Oxfordshire, pp 40–46

Gillam S 1999 Does the NHS need personal medical service pilots? They offer a test-bed for primary care trusts (editorial). British Medical Journal 318(7194):1302–1303

Harrison J, Redpath L 1998 Career start in County Durham. In: Harrison J, van Zwanenberg T (eds) GP Tomorrow. Radcliffe Medical Press, Abingdon, Oxfordshire, pp 59–75

NHS Executive 1996 Creative career paths in the NHS. NHS Executive, Leeds

NHS Executive 1998 The new NHS: modern and dependable. Developing primary care groups. (HSC 1998/129.) NHS Executive, Leeds

Primeline 2001 Primeline – everything you wanted to know about primary care management but did not know who to ask. Online. Available: www.primeline.org.uk

18 Managing information in general practice

Jeannette Naish

Most patients seeing a GP within the UK NHS now have to share their consultations with a third party present in the form of the doctor's computer. The keyboard, mouse and screen on the doctor's desk probably appeared without notice and without patients' permission for their personal details to be held in this way. How the computer changes the dynamics of the GP consultation will depend on how it is used by individual doctors, but there is no doubt that some difference must be made by its involvement in the consultation process.

L Most of the consultation models in current use were developed before the widespread advent of the computer introduced a 'third party' into the consultation. How do you think the various models would need to be modified to take account of this? What 'rules of etiquette' would you adopt for using the computer while the patient is present?

Until recently it was unlikely that GPs had any specific training on how to manage a face-to-face encounter with a patient and use a clinical computer system at the same time. With increasingly computer-based record keeping, skills are needed so that we can retrieve and enter data whilst still maintaining good communication with the patient.

Developing information technology has changed practice, and the profession now needs to consider the implications. There is no question that technological advances should improve overall patient care. But each practice must give careful consideration as to how these powerful systems can most efficiently and effectively be incorporated into their work such that they do provide the improvement in service and justify the cost and time taken in developing and running them. Most developments in clinical information technology (IT) have been led by technology rather than clinical need. The original Exeter System for general practice was developed for administrative purposes, for example, to monitor patient registrations and capitation payments. The concept was later adapted for clinical purposes. It does not need too much imagination to see that these are two very different kinds of functions and that the needs of the clinical users might be complex, particularly as they also directly involve patients.

These two main purposes for information management in general practice – administrative and clinical – will now be discussed.

Managing administrative information in practice

IT has revolutionised information for practice management (see also Chapter 17). The various administrative functions of a practice computer system can be summarised as follows.

Patient-related functions

- Maintaining a patient database – the age/sex register, new patient registrations and patient removals.
- Managing demand – appointments, home visits, out-of-hours activity and the administration of call/recall for chronic disease management, preventive programmes such as immunisations (all ages) and screening.
- Ensuring items of service claims and performance targets – this overlaps with the clinical side of the database where clinical activity, such as cervical cytology screening or clinical processes for chronic disease management, is recorded.

Practice-related functions

- Employed staff payroll, rotas, leave and contracts.
- Managing practice premises, running costs, maintenance, insurance and so on.
- Doctors' rotas and leave, out-of-hours arrangements.
- Book keeping, banking and petty cash.

Direct links with the Health Authority or Primary Care Trust improve efficiency in processing patient registrations and performance targets.

Validation of data becomes easier and payments can be processed more quickly.

Managing clinical information in practice

A wide variety of computer systems have been developed for use in general practice. All aim to help GPs to record and access clinical information and to make better decisions. As well as managing information on patients, computers allow us rapid access to a wealth of information from other sources, such as online textbooks, research databases and clinical decision systems. The following is an attempt to review briefly the clinical role of computers in general practice. The challenge is to enable enthusiasts to reflect in more depth and to encourage newcomers to think about what they would like a computer to do for them. The intention is to stimulate reflection about issues such as whether all practices should maintain a partially paper-based system or be moving towards 'paperless' patient records, rather than to advocate one system or another.

> **L** Widespread use of IT can bring access to enormous resources of clinical information within the reach of the patient as well as the doctor. What do you think could be the effects of this?

Record of patient encounters

The medical record of each patient is not only a record of separate episodes of contact with the GP but also a means of communicating information to others concerned with looking after the patient. Ideally, it will form a coherent lifelong medical and sometimes personal history. Symptoms of illness, diagnostic labels, measures of management processes and so on are not the only things that are important to know about a patient to provide good medical care.

Types of clinical data

The presenting complaint   The principle recognised by most experienced doctors that 'most diagnoses can be made on history alone' is no less true today in spite of the wealth of diagnostic aids and tests that are now available. The complex 'narrative' of any but the simplest complaint cannot be easily encapsulated in a computerised record. General practitioners are on the whole selective about what they record of what the patient says. Would the doctor's behaviour be the same whether writing a paper record or entering data on a computer? What would be missed out? Which would take longer?

The past medical history   A chronological summary of the medical problems that a patient has suffered is easily coded (always assuming that coding is systematic and consistent between doctors and between practices), stored on computer and retrieved. Similarly, a known family history could also be recorded. Medical problems of other members of the family registered with the same GP would also be easy to track. Social class, social problems, support and dysfunctional relationships would be less easy and not usually recorded, although they have a major influence on how people cope with illness, and on the quality of their lives.

The clinical examination   We see the findings from clinical examination as corroboration of the findings from the patient interview (history taking), to reduce uncertainty in clinical decisions. Not all clinical findings have a measurable value in the way that blood pressure or peak flow rates do. 'Looks ill' (or well) could be the clinical finding that determines whether the patient is advised to 'wait and see' or sent straight to hospital. So these need to be recorded as evidence to justify a clinical decision. How much of this can be coded and computerised?

Evaluation of findings   In an extreme case where we might be held to account for a clinical decision that went wrong and were required to justify our decision on the evidence of the patient's history and clinical findings, we would need to say how the jigsaw was put together: how each piece was evaluated in its own right and in relation to all the other pieces. Think how often a note is made in the margin of a paper record, which had a meaning at the time and was important for the final decision. Could the same be done easily on a computer? How much would it matter?

The action taken   The act of making a decision is included here: whether to investigate, give advice, make a diagnosis, give a prescription or refer on to somebody else (including someone in the practice, such as the nurse or counsellor). Most of the time, the consultation in general practice does not end with a diagnosis, but all this information about what action was taken can be coded, and would be useful and easily stored and retrieved. However, coding the information is not straightforward, with diagnostic labels probably being the trickiest.

Prescribing is in a different category and the computer is universally recognised as effective, particularly in repeat prescribing. It is possible to reduce errors, control the range of medicines used and, if prescribing protocols are operated consistently and diligently, monitor and review patients on long-term medication. Direct links with local pharmacists are also an advantage.

The patient outcome   Patient outcomes are not always easy to define. Death is unequivocal but is a blood pressure measurement an outcome? Patient outcomes would be important and useful to record and computerise for ease of storage and retrieval providing these are clearly defined, and the coding agreed and applied consistently.

Discussion points   ■ Consider what items of patient information you would or would not record on the computer. Consider what the computer is good for and what it is not.

- Review the different types of information recorded about patients in your own practice and reflect on other ways you might record each category.
- Reflect upon the costs and benefits of computerised records in relation to paper records.
- Compare the content and meaning of information recorded on paper records with computerised records. If you decide that you need both paper and computerised records, what would you record in each so as not to duplicate everything.
- What kind of information about patients would you share routinely with other agencies? Think about social services, the police, schools, insurance agencies and so on, as well as health services.

Aids to decision-making and templates based on clinical guidelines/protocols

Computer software for decision-making trees, or algorithms, have been developed for general practice to help us ensure that each step in the process of patient management is followed. Some are aimed at downward pressure on cost, for example, 'referral guidelines' in the USA were developed primarily for cost containment. Early research on whether these are useful for improving patient outcomes indicate that they have a favourable effect on identifying new cases and on follow-up, but are much less conclusive about whether physician knowledge and patient management are better. Of course, it can also be argued that identifying unmet need and preventing, or reducing, risk factors would increase demand and cost.

PRODIGY is a national initiative to develop a computerised decision support system for UK general practice. Prescribing has been a major focus. Further information can be obtained from the PRODIGY website (www.prodigy.nhs.uk).

Templates for specific conditions are very useful aids for recording the procedures carried out during a patient encounter. These are generally based on evidence-based guidelines. There still remains the issue of the patient narrative during these encounters; whether and how this should be recorded.

Morbidity register: audit of performance

If diagnostic and patient outcome information were systematically and consistently coded, and stored, then the patient database could be used as a morbidity register. The operative words are systematic and consistent. The Read system of clinical coding is widely used in general practice in the UK but is not compatible with some other forms of disease coding, such as the International Disease Codes system. Clarity is also needed for distinction between process of care, outcome or diagnostic label.

Data stored in a database of patient morbidity could easily be retrieved to examine disease incidence and prevalence; audit processes of care against agreed guidelines and, when possible, monitor outcomes. A practice mortality register would also be useful, but not so easy to set up.

Service activity could also be thought of as patient outcomes, such as diagnosis specific emergency hospital admissions, attendance at Accident and Emergency Departments, elective hospital admissions, referrals to social services or community health services among others. Private- and voluntary-sector referrals could also be included.

Discussion points

- How would you set up a practice mortality register?
- What patient outcomes would be important for measuring the effectiveness of particular chronic disease management programmes?

The practice computer as a means of communication

Electronic networking is increasingly available in health care. Much of it will help to improve the efficiency in service delivery, and sometimes to improve the quality of patient care. NHSnet is now accessible to all general practices and provides the possibility of communication between all NHS services. Possible links with other systems could be briefly summarised to perform the following functions:

- Links for investigations (path, radiology, etc.) – need to be reliable and secure; links with other clinicians (nurses, health visitors, consultants, pharmacists, etc.) also need to be reliable and secure.
- Links with administrative systems at Health Authorities, Primary Care Trusts – reliability and efficiency are essential.
- Links with other agencies – social services, police, etc. must conform with data protection legislation. Data protection issues abound in this area.
- Links with patients – also patient information, quality of patient information and access. If patients are truly to be active participants in decisions about their health care, then the information they are given must be accurately based on current best evidence, and be acceptable and useful. There is anecdotal evidence of the proliferation of poor quality information for patients.
- Access and retrieval of 'evidence' at the point of use for GPs engaged in patient care – sources include textbooks, the internet, databases for published research and relevant peer-reviewed journals. This requirement is very different to that for researchers. Current information retrieval systems are primarily designed for research rather than clinical users. Although decision support software is an attempt at redressing this mismatch, the design, implementation and critical evaluation of retrieval systems for clinical care should be guided by the needs of clinical users.

The details for every aspect of information management cannot be fully explored here. It is suggested that you take a little time, with your colleagues, to reflect upon:

- how different practices make use of these advances in communication technology

- how effective and useful these links are
- whether there is a standard for the most effective use for this.

Use of anonymous, aggregate clinical data for public health purposes

There is a wealth of demographic and morbidity data in general practice, which could be used for assessing need for resources in the population. This in turn could be evidence to inform service planning and resource distribution. The challenge is in the reliability and quality of these data, and how they could be accessed. The Computerised Health Data in General Practice (CHDGP) project used the MIQUEST approach for extracting aggregated, anonymous clinical patient data from volunteered general practice computer systems. Such a software system is needed because there are so many general practice systems in use, which are incompatible with each other. The second problem is the reliability and quality of data, in that not all practices code and record patient information, nor do they consistently use agreed, common coding systems. This has evolved into the Primary Care Information System (PRIMIS), which is based at the University of Nottingham and provides help on the most effective use of GP computer systems, managing and retrieving data, analysis of aggregated data and audit feedback (www.primis. nottingham.ac.uk).

User requirements for general practice systems

The challenges facing information technology in general practice are both conceptual and technical. Most of the difficulties with general practice clinical information management are the result of failure to acknowledge and define the conceptual challenges.

Listed below are some issues relevant to clinical users of general practice computing systems. They are not exhaustive but might serve to enable reflection on what you, as a clinical user, might want to specify as the basic purposes and value of the systems to inform the technical experts:

- Security will always be a source of controversy when sensitive personal data are being recorded and stored electronically without the permission of the subject: the patient. This might be breached externally, or internally by authorised staff (including doctors) misusing sensitive information. All practices must be registered under the Data Protection Act and follow the guidance it provides.
- Reliability and validity are key goals for patient information. For example, disease coding could be checked using other parameters, such as prescribing, information from other sources, such as consultant letters, and some process measures, such as blood glucose levels for diabetes. Proper comparisons of reliability between systems are harder but it might be possible to compare 'down' times between systems.
- Access to practice data (NHSnet, PRIMIS, etc.) – the issues of data protection are paramount. It should also be remembered that, as well as the patient, the practice is also the data subject. The integrity and

reliability of the data is once more at issue. The 'membership' for access to practice data needs defining.

■ Sustainability – general practice has been going through major change since the early 1980s. In a changing environment, with constant change in use, can the system adapt to changing use or does the user have to adapt to the limitations of the system and progress in technologies?

■ Cost-effectiveness – is the system more effective (meets all the purposes for which a patient record is intended) and cheaper (time and money) than existing (paper) systems? What is the evidence?

Summary

■ Almost all general practices in the UK are now computerised to a greater or lesser extent.

■ IT has revolutionised much of the administration of general practice. For many, it has also had dramatic effects on direct clinical care, with increasing numbers of practices moving to paperless record systems.

■ Electronic communication is the current area of growth, aided by developments such as health authority and pathology links and NHSnet.

■ The impact of the computer in the GP consultation is an area in need of further research.

L One further area into which IT is bound to expand is the assessment of medical knowledge and competence. The MRCGP is currently exploring ways of computerising parts of the examination. Bearing in mind what this chapter has to say about the recording of 'narrative', do you think this would be progress?

Further reading

Gardner M 1997 Information retrieval for patient care. British Medical Journal 314:950

Gray J, Majeed A, Kerry S, Rowlands G 2000 Identifying patients with ischaemic heart disease in general practice: cross sectional study of paper and computerised medical records. British Medical Journal 321:548–550

Keen J, Wyatt J 2000 Back to basics on the NHS networking. British Medical Journal 321:875–878

Montgomery A, Fahey T 1998 A systematic review of the use of computers in the management of hypertension. Journal of Epidemiology and Community Health 52:520–525

Preece J 2000 The use of computers in general practice. Churchill Livingstone, London

Useful contacts

PRODIGY
www.prodigy.nhs.uk

Primary Care Information System, University of Nottingham
www.primis.nottingham.ac.uk

SECTION 6

Further reading and sources of information

Further reading and sources of information

Joe Rosenthal, Surinder Singh

The registrar year is the end of the beginning of education for general practice. Where do we go from here? The breadth and rate of change in the discipline make it essential that we continue to learn throughout our working lives. But learning is not simply the acquisition of knowledge, and continuing education is not just 'keeping up to date'. We need to carry on learning to remain stimulated and enjoy our work. In this way we benefit not only ourselves but our patients and colleagues.

Numerous and varied learning opportunities are available to us in forms as diverse as books, journals, magazines, audiotapes, videotapes, DVDs, CD-ROMs, websites, seminars, practitioners' groups, lectures and courses. However, with all the old and new technology available to us, the most valuable sources of learning remain our colleagues and our patients in day-to-day practice.

The list of sources that follows is presented as a 'menu' to sample according to your taste and appetite. Please also see the reference and further reading lists provided at the end of each chapter.

General reading

Berger J, Mohr P 1967 A fortunate man. Penguin, London

Cronin AJ 1939 The citadel. Gollancz, London (republished 1996 by Orion, London)

Greenhalgh P, Hurwitz B 1998 Narrative based medicine. BMJ Books, London

Helman CG 1984 Culture, health and illness. Wright, London

Huygen FJA 1978 Family medicine: the medical life history of families. Dekker & Vandervegt, Nijmegen, Netherlands (republished 1990 by the RCGP)

McWhinney IR 1989 A textbook of family medicine. Oxford University Press, Oxford

Munthe A 1929 The story of San Michele. John Murray, London (republished 1990 by Flamingo, London)

Stacey E 2000 Hot topics in general practice. BIOS Scientific Publishers Ltd, Oxford

Stephenson A 1998 A textbook of general practice. Arnold, London

Stott P 1983 Milestones. Pan, London (republished 1991 by the RCGP)

Widgery D 1992 Some lives! A GP's East End. Sinclair Stevenson, London

GP training/summative assessment and MRCGP examination

Abrams W, Howell S 2002 The GP registrar survival guide. BIOS Scientific Publishers Ltd, Oxford

Gardiner P, Chana N, Jones R 2001 An insider's guide to the MRCGP oral exam. Radcliffe Medical Press, Abingdon, Oxfordshire

Hall M, Dwyer D, Lewis T 1999 The GP training handbook. Blackwell Science, Oxford

Moore R 2000 The MRCGP examination: a guide for candidates and teachers, 4th edn. The Royal College of General Practitioners, London

Palmer K T 1997 Notes for the MRCGP, 3rd edn. Blackwell Science, Oxford

Skelton J, Field S, Wiskin C, Tate P 1998 Those things you say ... consultation skills and the MRCGP examination. Radcliffe Medical Press, Abingdon, Oxfordshire

Vocational Training Summative Assessment Board 1998 Protocol for the management of summative assessment: statement by the Joint Committee on Postgraduate Training for General Practice. RCGP, London

The consultation

Balint M 1957 The doctor, his patient and the illness. Tavistock Publications, London

Byrne PS, Long BEL 1976 Doctors talking to patients. HMSO, London

Heron J 1975 Six category intervention analysis. Human Potential Resource Group, Guildford

Kurtz S, Silverman J, Draper J 1998 Teaching and learning communication skills in medicine. Radcliffe Medical Press, Abingdon, Oxfordshire

Neighbour R 1987 The inner consultation. Petroc Press, Newbury

Pendleton D, Schofield T, Tate P, Havelock P 1984 The consultation: an approach to learning and teaching. Oxford University Press, Oxford

RCGP 2002 MRCGP Examination Regulations & Video Assessment of Consulting Skills Workbook. The Examination Department, Royal College of General Practitioners, London

Silverman J, Kurtz S, Draper J 1998 Skills for communicating with patients. Radcliffe Medical Press, Abingdon, Oxfordshire

Tate P 1994 The doctor's communication handbook. Radcliffe Medical Press, Abingdon, Oxfordshire

Epidemiology, evidence-based medicine and statistics

Bland M 2000 An introduction to medical statistics. Oxford Medical Publications, London

Greenhalgh T 2000 How to read a paper. BMJ Publications, London

Jones R, Kinmonth AL 1995 A critical reading for primary care. Oxford University Press, Oxford

Morrell D 1988 Epidemiology in general practice. Oxford University Press, Oxford

Petrie A, Sabin C 2000 Medical statistics at a glance. Blackwell Science, Oxford

Ridsdale L 1995 Evidence-based general practice: a critical reader. WB Saunders, London

Ridsdale L (ed) 1998 Evidence-based practice in primary care. Churchill Livingstone, London

Sackett D, Hayes RB, Guyatt GH, Tugwell P 1991 Clinical epidemiology: a basic science for clinical medicine. Little, Brown, Boston

Sackett DL, Richardson WS, Rosenberg WMC, Haynes RB 2000 Evidence-based medicine: how to practise and teach EBM, 2nd edn. Churchill Livingstone, London

Silagy C, Haines A 2001 Evidence based practice in primary health care. BMJ Publications, London

Medical ethics

Beauchamp TL, Childress JF 1994 Principles of medical ethics, 4th edn. Oxford University Press, Oxford

British Medical Association 1993 Medical ethics today: its practice and philosophy. BMA Publications, London

Campbell A, Gillett G, Jones G 2001 Medical ethics. Oxford University Press, Oxford

Gillon R 1995 Philosophical medical ethics. Wiley, Chichester

Leung W-C 2000 Law for doctors. Blackwell Science, Oxford

Mason JK, McCall Smith RA 1994 Law and medical ethics. Butterworths, London

Orme-Smith A, Spicer J 2001 Ethics in general practice. Radcliffe Medical Press, Abingdon, Oxfordshire

Toon P 1999 Towards a philosophy of general practice: a study of the virtuous practitioner. RCGP Occasional Paper 78. RCGP, London

Practice management

Bolden K, Lewis A, Sawyer B 1992 Practice management. Blackwell Science, Oxford

Dean J 2000 Making sense of practice finance. Radcliffe Medical Press, Abingdon, Oxfordshire

Ellis N, Chisholm J 1997 Making sense of the red book, 3rd edn. Radcliffe Medical Press, Abingdon, Oxfordshire

Hasler J, Bryceland C, Hobden-Clarke L, Moreton P 1991 Handbook of practice management. Churchill Livingstone, London

Audit and research

Armstrong D, Grace J 2000 Research methods and audit in general practice. Oxford General Practice Series, Oxford

Carter Y, Shaw S, Thomas C (eds) 2000 Master classes in primary care research. The Royal College of General Practitioners, London

Carter Y, Thomas C 1996 Research methods in primary care. Radcliffe Medical Press, Abingdon, Oxfordshire

Howie JGR 1989 Research in general practice, 2nd edn. Chapman & Hall, London

Lawrence M, Schofield T (eds) 1993 Medical audit in primary health care. Oxford General Practice Series, Oxford

Marinker M 1995 Audit and general practice. BMJ Books, London

Social sciences

Armstrong D 1995 An outline of sociology as applied to medicine. Butterworth-Heinemann, Oxford

Ogden J 2000 Health psychology. A textbook. Open University Press, Buckingham

Scambler G 1997 Sociology as applied to medicine. Saunders, London

Weinmann J 1987 An outline of psychology as applied to medicine. Butterworth-Heinemann, Oxford

Some useful websites

The internet provides an enormous range of information on all aspects of health and health services. There are numerous official and unofficial sites available on moreorless any topic. It is important, though, to be aware that most sites are not currently subject to formal quality control of any kind. Be aware that anyone can post a web page and that information even on official sites is not always up-to-date or accurate. Having said all this it is hard to imagine now how we would manage without this rich mine of information. The sites listed below are all active at time of writing and, in our opinion, worth referring to when needed. We would also recommend the 2002 BMJ article dedicated to this new and 'transformational' way of communicating: *Trust me I'm a website* British Medical Journal 2002 324(7337):555–622, 9 March 2002.

General information for the clinician

www.bandolier.com: useful evidence-based health care newsletter.

www.doctors.net.uk: a website for practising doctors (i.e. those registered with the GMC) with online information in textbooks, the Cochrane database, Medline and travel information.

www.doh.gov.uk/: the address for the general department of health website. Since it is so large you need time and patience. However, it is very comprehensive.

www.doh.gov.uk/cmoconsult1.htm: website for the document *Supporting Doctors, Protecting Patients* (Department of Health).

www.doh.gov.uk/ipu/strategy/nsf/3.htm: a website for the best use of information technology in cardiac care and the NHS plan.

www.doh.gov.uk/pricare/fees.htm: the site that states the revised fees and allowances payable to general practitioners in England and Wales.

www.dpp.org.uk: a website for the charity doctor–patient partnership (DPP). The DPP is a UK charity which aims to facilitate a two-way communication between patients and doctors.

www.drsdesk.sghms.ac.uk/: The 'Doctors Desk' project is developing a front end to various sources of information (ebm, practice guidelines, databases, e-mail, the NHSNet) and the means to open practice and hospital computer systems, for GPs. Currently being tested in STaRNet (South Thames Region's Research Network).

www.nelh.nhs.uk: the Primary Care National Electronic Library for Health Programme – working towards developing a digital library for NHS staff, patients and the public.

www.nhsdirect.nhs.uk: a general website for general information about all health – this also contains a searchable database of conditions and treatments.

www.omni.ac.uk/browse/mesh/detail/C0015607L00 15607.html: OMNI provides links to several primary-care-related websites.

www.primis.nottingham.ac.uk/: this website, based at the University of Nottingham, provides help on the most effective use of GP computer systems, managing and retrieving data, analysis of aggregated data and audit feedback.

www.prodigy.nhs.uk: this is a national initiative to develop a computerised decision support system for UK general practice. Prescribing has been a major focus up to now.

www.update-software.com/Cochrane/default.htm: The Cochrane Library – a source of reliable information on the effects of healthcare interventions.

www.york.ac.uk/inst/crd: website for the *Effective Health Care Bulletin*, providing access to a rolling programme of systematic reviews.

Education and training

www.bmjcareers.com: website for those who want advice on career options.

www.doctoronline.nhs.uk: the website for the National Office for Summative Assessment.

www.doh.gov.uk/cmo/cmoh.htm: a website for the Chief Medical Officer's update for general practitioners and all NHS staff.

www.doh.gov.uk/gpappraisal: the Department of Health website for GP appraisal and how it links with re-validation.

www.hda-online.org.uk: a special health authority that aims to improve the health of people in England – especially those groups who suffer from problems related to health inequalities.

www.jcptgp.org.uk: website for the Joint Committee on Postgraduate training in general practice.

www.londondeanery.ac.uk/home.htm: the website for the London Deanery, where details of summative assessment guide is available.

www.medirect.com/professional-development/: a website for professional handbook training.

www.primeline.org.uk: Primeline is a site for practice managers; basically it is 'everything you wanted to know about Primary Care Management but did not know who to ask'.

www.rcog.org.uk: the website for the Royal College of Obstetricians and Gynaecologists.

www.rcpch.org.uk: the website for the Royal College of Paediatrics and Child Health.

www.rcplondon.ac.uk: the website for the Royal College of Physicians.

www.roysocmed.ac.uk: the website for the Royal Society of Medicine.

www.rcgp.org.uk: the website for the Royal College of General Practitioners.

Journals

Many journals now have at least partial access available online. These are just a selection of those directly relevant to UK general practice. Many more can be accessed, e.g. by links from OMNI:

www.bmj.com: British Medical Journal.

www.fampract.oupjournals.org/: Family Practice.

www.lancet.com: the Lancet.

www.priory.com/gp.htm: General Practice On Line.

www.rcgp.org.uk/rcgp/journal/index.asp: British Journal of General Practice.

The National Health Service

www.archive.official-documents.co.uk/document/doh/newnhs/contents.htm: website for *The New NHS: modern, dependable.* HMSO, London.

www.clinical-governance.com: a bulletin published by the Royal Society of Medicine around clinical governance issues and clinical risk management.

www.dhsspsni.gov.uk: website for NHS – Northern Ireland, i.e. Department of Health, Social Services and Public Safety in Northern Ireland.

www.doh.gov.uk: website for the Department of Health.

www.doh.gov.uk/newnhs/quality.htm: website for *A First Class Service: Quality in the new NHS.* HMSO, London.

www.doh.gov.uk/nhscomplaintsreform/evaluation report.pdf: a report on the evaluation of complaints procedure in the NHS in England and Wales.

www.doh.gov.uk/nsc/index.htm: website for the National Screening Committee.

www.doh.gov.uk/nshs/summary.htm: the website for the Department of Health National Sexual Health Strategy, initially published in the summer of 2001.

www.doh.gov.uk/pricare/clingov.htm: this website is about clinical governance and is accessible through the generic DoH site.

www.dwp.gov.uk: website for the Department for Work and Pensions.

www.nhsatoz.org: website for the A–Z of the NHS in terms of provision, services and where to go.

www.nhsdirect.nhs.uk: website for NHS Direct helpline.

www.nhs.uk: website for the general NHS.

www.nhs.uk/nationalplan: website for *The NHS Plan. A plan for investment, a plan for reform.*

www.nhs.uk/zerotolerance: website for the NHS campaign Zero tolerance re: violence in work.

www.ombudsman.org.uk/hse/index.html: the website for the NHS ombudsman – his office investigates complaints within the NHS.

www.show.scot.nhs.uk: website for NHS – Scotland.

www.show.scot.nhs.uk/publications/me/complaints/: the equivalent of the above report, but for Scotland.

www.wales.nhs.uk: website for NHS – Wales.

Other organisations

www.bma.org.uk: the British Medical Association – hard at work on several fronts, including negotiations on a new contract.

www.chi.nhs.uk: the site for the Commission for Health Improvement.

www.gmc-uk.org: the General Medical Council – based in London but may be having at least one other regional office in Manchester, UK.

www.helpdoctor.co.uk/sick_doctors.htm: National Counselling Service for Sick Doctors. A confidential, independent advisory service for sick doctors supported by the BMA and the medical royal colleges.

www.kingsfund.org.uk: the King's Fund is an independent charitable foundation whose goal is to improve health, especially in London.

www.lmc.org.uk: the site for the London-wide Local Medical Committees.

www.the-mdu.com: this defence organisation has a new website including multiple FAQs, general information and what to do in a crisis. Free teaching pack for GP registrars on medical ethics and law also available.

www.mps.org.uk: website for the Medical Protection Society.

www.nagpc.org.uk: website for the National Association of GP Co-operatives.

www.nanp.org.uk: the National Association of Non-Principals (very good information including education and training).

www.nice.org.uk: the site dedicated to NICE – the National Institute for Clinical Excellence.

www.npsa.org.uk: National Patient Safety Agency – established in 2002 in respect of the new culture within the NHS about learning from mistakes and anticipating their occurrence.

www.ons.gov.uk: the site for the Office of National Statistics.

www.phls.co.uk/facts/index.htm: an excellent website for those interested in public health issues – this one contains a list of facts and figures about many conditions.

www.rcgp.org.uk: The Royal College of General Practitioners – responsible for the exams and much else.

www.sick-doctors-trust.co.uk: the Sick Doctors Trust provides advice and treatment for doctors suffering from addiction to alcohol or other drugs.

www.tht.org.uk: Terence Higgins Trust, a prominent UK-based HIV/AIDS charity providing specialist advice on issues related to HIV and AIDS.

Prescribing

www.bnf.org: the website for the British National Formulary.

www.mca.gov.uk: the Committee on Safety of Medicines/Medicines Control Agency.

www.mca.gov.uk/ourwork/monitorsafequalmed/currentproblems/currentproblems.htm: a list of the current drug problems come to light.

www.medical-devices.gov.uk: the Medical Devices Agency.

www.npc.co.uk: website for the National Treatment Centre – responsible for MeReC, a national newsletter providing up-to-date information on drugs for clinicians, including for general practitioners.

www.ppa.org.uk: website for the Prescription Pricing Authority.

www.which.net/health/dtbtreatment.html: the website for the Drugs and Therapeutics bulletin – a very useful source of advice and guidance.

Index

Notes: Page numbers in *italics* refer to tables, figures or boxed materials. *vs.* indicates a comparison.

Abortion Act (1967), 165, 170
access
    information management, 227–228
    to medical care *see* National Health Service (NHS)
    as performance indicator, *109*
    to records *see* access to records
Access to Medical Records Act (AHRA) (1990), 188
Access to Medical Reports Act (1988), 188
access to records, 187–190
    Access to Health Records Act (1990), 188
    Access to Medical Reports Act (1988), 188
    Caldicott Report, 189
    case studies, 188–189
    consent, 188
    The Data Protection Act (1998), 187
    information given, 187
    mental health, 189
    NHS Plan 2001, 188
    post-mortem, 189
    procedure, 187
    withholding of, 187–188
    see also confidentiality; patient records
accidents, disease prevention, 91
accountability, clinical governance, 107, 113
active euthanasia, *163*
active listening, health education, 99
adjustment phase, 8–10
adolescents
    access to records, 188–189

consent, 175–176
disease prevention, *90*
adults
    disease prevention, *90*
    screening, *95*
advance directives, 175
adverse event monitoring, clinical governance, 114
age discrimination, *83*
ageing *see* geriatric medicine
AIDS, 77, 80–81
    websites, 86–87
    see also HIV infections
alcohol-related illness, prevention, 91
anecdotal evidence, 118
annual reports, practice manager role, 213
antenatal clinics, 11
antenatal disease prevention, *90*
antenatal screening, *95*
anthropological model of illness, 63, 65–66
    in consultations, 64, *64*
antibiotics, sore throat therapy, 73–74
APC Journal Club, 124
appeals procedure, summative assessment failure, 26
assessments, clinical governance, 113
assisted suicide, *163*
audit, clinical *see* clinical audits
autonomy, 162, 167
    competence, 162
    mental problems, 176

baby clinics, 11
bad news, communication skills, 167
behaviour models
    consulting skills, 46–47
    of illness, 63
beneficence, 162, 168, 176

Best Evidence, 124
biomedical model of illness, 63
British Journal of General Practice, 8
    evidence-based medicine, 124
    MRCGP exam preparation, 40
British Medical Journal
    evidence-based medicine, 124
    MRCGP exam preparation, 40
British National Formulary, MRCGP exam preparation, 41
British Regional Heart Study, disease prevention, 94–95
building management, practice manager role, 214

Caldicott Report, access to records, 189
Calgary–Cambridge Observation Guide, 48
camera position, video recordings, 49–50
cancer, disease prevention, 91
case finding, 96
case law, 171
case studies
    access to records, 188–189
    clinical guidelines, 127–128
    confidentiality, 183–187
    evidence-based practice, 119–120
    geriatric medicine, 84–85
catalytic interventions, 47
cathartic interventions, 47
centralised appointment system, 6
Centre for Reviews and Dissemination, 124
cerebrovascular disease, disease prevention, 91
CHAIN (Contact, Help Advice and Information Network), 125
change promotion, health education, 100

237